HOUSE CALL

HOUSE CALL

UNDERSTANDING HOW
TELEMEDICINE IS POISED TO
TRANSFORM HEALTH CARE IN
RURAL AMERICA AND BEYOND

ANNA DACCACHE

NEW DEGREE PRESS

HOUSE CALL

Understanding How Telemedicine Is Poised to Transform Health Care in Rural America and Beyond

ISBN   978-1-63676-509-9   *Paperback*

978-1-63676-031-5   *Kindle Ebook*

978-1-63676-032-2   *Ebook*

Pour mon Jeddo, mon héros, you are infinitie. I am because of you.

CONTENTS

Of all the forms of inequality, injustice in health is the most shocking and inhuman.
—DR. MARTIN LUTHER KING, JR.

INTRODUCTION

———

"At three in the morning, [Public Safety] came into my hotel room to pack all my stuff because I was physically unable."

The first time Rachel (a pseudonym) told me her story, I remember being both shocked and angry.

We went to a school in rural Virginia. Late into our freshman year, my friend Rachel felt ill on her drive back to school after a break. She wasn't well enough to get back, so our school's public safety picked her up and brought her to our university health center. There, Rachel and the nurses on duty immediately recognized meningitis symptoms, something her sister had been diagnosed with several years prior. The staff immediately rushed her to the local hospital.

The care she received upon her arrival was less than adequate. Apart from the fact that the staff was more concerned with making Rachel—who was clearly in distress—pay her bill, the doctor on call at the time completely lacked any bedside manner. "They totally disregarded my sister's medical history and the fact that I quite obviously was showing signs of meningitis." When he finally got around to testing her after trying to diagnose her with an even rarer disease, it took eight attempts to conduct a lumbar puncture properly.

When recounting the story, Rachel visibly cringes as she thinks back on how her admitting doctor tried to conduct the spinal tap *seven* times before finally calling for the anesthesiologist to do it. The test came back positive for meningitis, so they sent her to UVA Medical Center in Charlottesville to receive care. She had to be admitted for long-term treatment, which was contrary to what the doctor at the first hospital had told her; he had argued she was well enough to go home.

To reiterate, the doctor was prepared to send a nineteen-year-old girl with meningitis back to her college dorm without a proper diagnosis, risking infection to countless other students and foregoing the lifesaving treatment she needed.

I'm telling you this story because it goes to show how resources, specialists, and even just being made to feel comfortable during a terrifying medical ordeal are completely lacking. And yes, the hospital and the doctor were at fault, but they also didn't know what to do in that situation because they'd never prepared for it. Had telemedicine been a part of her care and had the local hospital been able to call a specialist, maybe Rachel's whole ordeal could have been avoided.

It's time to consider how telemedicine is poised to transform our mental health and wellness care over the next decade. I shudder at the thought of what might have happened to Rachel had she not been properly diagnosed. I was scared for my friend and am scared for anyone who may face this kind of situation in the future. I am angry at the broken system that put her and so many others in such a compromising and vulnerable position. At the same time, I am also hopeful that we are on the cusp of entirely revolutionizing the access and quality of health care as we know it, through technology like telemedicine.

THE STATE OF AMERICAN HEALTH CARE

We have to look at the state of our society if we want to grow and move forward. About 20 percent—roughly one in five—adults in the United States live with mental illness.[1] Countless challenges are facing our health care systems, but the lack of adequate mental health treatment is a crucial one that we must address (an idea I explore further in Chapter 2). Unfortunately, our society is still struggling to regard mental illness as seriously as we view physical ailments, even though our mental well-being informs our physical well-being and vice versa. We must take both seriously because unfortunately, over 60 percent of rural Americans live in areas that have shortages of mental health professionals.[2] The fact that 90 percent of psychiatrists and psychologists are located in metropolitan areas means that a law enforcement officer is the most likely mental health crisis responder in rural America.[3] The system needs to change to better suit the needs of rural communities

---

1   National Institute of Mental Health, "Mental Illness," NIMH, Mental Illness, last modified February, 2019.

2   National Institute of Mental Health, "Mental Health and Rural America: Challenges and Opportunities." NIMH. Last modified May 28, 2018.

3   Ibid.

All of America—but particularly rural America—is suffering from a health crisis where unimaginable costs and a lack of access to proper resources plague communities. This is especially true in the case of treating mental illness, and that is the focus of my book: how to create a more community-based approach to health through telemedicine.[4] The laws surrounding telehealth are vague and outdated, so I dream that my book will start a dialogue about necessary policy changes that would allow state and local governments to work with hospitals and university health care systems to invest in and grow telemedicine practices. While some regulations have changed in light of COVID-19, the problem remains; we have no guarantee that the changes that adopted for the current reality will remain afterward.

Healthcare systems can apply and use telemedicine in various ways:

- Live video through a two-way audio-visual link between patient and provider
- Asynchronous video such as a recorded transmission of patient health history to a medical specialist
- Remote patient-monitoring using tools to record personal health and medical data in one place for review by the provider in a different place

---

4   Andy Blackwell, "Artificial Intelligence Meets Mental Health Therapy | Andy Blackwell | TEDxNatick – YouTube," TEDx Talks, uploaded March 11, 2020, YouTube video, 18:45.

- Mobile health, which is the accessing of public health and healthcare information through a mobile device[5]

We have so much to look forward to in the telemedicine space. Companies and universities in the United States and around the globe are developing programs, building platforms, and raising the bar for what we can expect from telemedicine. One such example is Texas A&M University's Telebehavioral Health program. What started in 2009 as just a way of working from their desks, Dr. Jim Burdine and Dr. Timothy Elliot have built a groundbreaking behavioral health program through the use of medicine that is fully integrated in the Brazos Valley communities in Texas. See chapter 8 for a more detailed account of the work the Telebehavioral Health Program has done.

THE NECESSARY COMPONENTS

We can take away three key components from the Texas A&M example: accessibility, collaboration/cooperation, and community integration. Small communities often lack the resources and professionals to provide necessary care, particularly when it comes to addressing mental health. Building programs or systems that make accessing care easier for these communities would allow for healthier, happier, and safer towns. It is both medical innovation at its finest and a return to community health as it used to be.

---

5   Office of the National Coordinator for Health Information Technology, "Telemedicine and Telehealth," Health Information Technology. Last modified September 24, 2020 .

When thinking about improving outcomes in and providing access to rural areas, telemedicine is a clear solution. Many think telemedicine is an interesting option but believe it's not necessarily a major solution; they view it more as a nice addition. However, telemedicine can and will transform the medical industry, especially with respect to access to mental health care, but even across the board. Why? One must consider the communities, like Plentywood, Montana, that are home to only 1,700 people and almost an hour away from the nearest hospital. While an idyllic town, Plentywood, like many other rural communities, lacks the mental health providers and other specialists that are more readily available in more populous areas. Telemedicine can help remove the barriers to care for people living in areas such as Plentywood that lack comprehensive medical coverage or for people who don't have transportation to and from medical care.[6] Telemedicine has a clear potential to completely change how we approach medicine and health care in the future.

*****

I have often asked myself and those around me why small towns do not have the same kind of medical specialists available in metropolitan or even suburban areas. This is both a simple and wildly complex question and issue. You have to account for the fact that a primary care physician or dentist living in small-town Montana is much more likely to build a practice there. However, within specialized

---

6   Centers for Disease Control and Prevention, "Telehealth in Rural Communities," National Center for Chronic Disease Prevention and Health Promotion, CDC, last modified August 18, 2020.

fields—particularly trauma medicine and mental illness—professionals find it more difficult to sustain a career in small towns because it is almost impossible to have a large enough client base or to not burnout from being the only one available. Despite this challenge, we cannot let these communities fall to the wayside. We cannot let them not have necessary care. Fortunately, institutions of higher learning, health care companies, and tech companies are demonstrating how telemedicine can fill the gap by connecting the more rural and isolated hospitals to premier care specialists.

Health tech companies are in a unique position to disrupt the health care industry and promote positive change with the development of platforms that could make accessing care so much easier. For example, the summer after my junior year of college, I interned at a health tech startup focused on making mental health care more affordable and accessible to everyone. Our client base was exclusively individuals on Medicare or Medicaid. Realizing that structural change in health care was seemingly so unreachable was simultaneously a devastating yet motivating experience for me. While my interest in bettering mental health treatment has always existed, this experience inspired my passion for transforming American health care, and thus led to the birth of this book. The endless research I performed during my internship forced me to confront the reality of the health outcomes in different parts of the country. Further, the interviews I conducted with politicians and medical and tech professionals combined with my own experiences and vested interest in telemedicine uniquely situates me to write this book.

I learned that when you break it down, our communities have an unimaginable number of people with mental illness—most of them on Medicaid—that are not able to get treatment because it is neither accessible nor affordable. After this realization, I adjusted my educational and job plans; I am now working on a Master of Science degree in Computer Science with a specialization in data science and artificial intelligence so that I can pursue a career at the intersection of health care and technology. I have a specific interest in mobilizing telemedicine as a way to transform access to care and improve health outcomes.

This book serves to explore how medical treatment has evolved and how its evolution has led to a reliance on hospitals, which has left many behind. We must analyze how we have gotten to where we are today in order to understand the steps we need to take to improve health outcomes for rural communities and beyond. We need to take a proactive approach to health care as opposed to a reactive one. In this book, I will dig into what telemedicine is and how it can transform our approach to health care—particularly mental illness. I also hope to unpack the barriers to entry for rural communities and introduce the principles of the much-needed telemedicine mental health revolution, as well as determine who should lead the charge and how we can accelerate it.

This book paints a picture of the stark reality facing rural Americans today when it comes to mental health and access to care. We should all care about this because a healthier community means a safer, happier, and more productive community. Our health and the health of others inform the world around us. On the surface, a book about health care and telemedicine may come across as daunting, dense, tedious, or all of the above. I know that I felt that way when I initially started writing the book, but I focused my approach to make this a book for everyone. If we, as a society, can better understand the myriad ways in which our systems of health can be improved upon, we can contribute. You don't have to be a doctor to do so; this is a book for not only mental health professionals, health-tech innovators, and politicians, but also for everyone else.

I believe that integration is key. A community is only as effective as the sum of its parts, and for health care and, by extension, telemedicine to work, we all need to understand it.

My hope is that by reading this book you will not only feel like you have a better grasp of our health care system as a whole and how different it looks across the country, but that you also will become more aware of the already existing products, systems, and institutions that try to combat the lack of accessibility and affordability that makes health care so daunting of an obstacle to tackle.

CHAPTER 1

IN THE BEGINNING

It was 2:00 a.m. on a Saturday in March during my sopho-more year of college. I was fast asleep in bed when some girls I lived with barged into my room. The cacophony of their voices shouting what I interpreted as nonsense woke me up. I groggily tried to follow along with what they were trying to tell me after they switched on the harsh light.

Finally, one of them got the message out in a rush, her words tripping over themselves: "Anna, Anna… she's unconscious. They sent her to the hospital." I was now wide awake.

We cannot imagine a world without hospitals. I mean, what is medical care without them? Health care in the United States is almost completely centered around reactionary care. Professionals often preach the importance of preventative health, but our reliance on emergency services in times of crisis or even just uncertainty says otherwise.

In direct response to emergency rooms (ER) being over-crowded, urgent care (UC) clinics were adopted. While these are not devoid of value—they are an essential part of responding to crises and trauma—people often show up to the ER or UC because they don't know where else to go, not because they need to be there. Could medicine as we know it exist without these institutions? Maybe, maybe not, but I do know that we need structural change to improve access to and outcomes of care, particularly when considering health care on an integrated level that incorporates both physical and mental care.

So, what did American medicine look like before the growth of the hospital system? In the sixteenth, seventeenth, and even well into the eighteenth centuries, doctors weren't just doctors. They were preachers, politicians, or an amalgamation of other professions, which we can see in the "preacher-physician" of Colonial New England. Although not wholly unheard of in present-day Western culture, the idea of a spiritual leader acting as a medical professional would, for many, be confusing, concerning, and inadequate. In Colonial New England, where faith was the foundation of society and permeated every aspect of life, preachers oversaw medical treatment because "illness was linked to original and personal sin."[7] Puritan leaders in New England often ascribed widespread sickness to God's will as a sort of punishment attributed to their collective sin.[8] However, as more and more people came from Europe to settle in what is now the United States, the religious and cultural landscape shifted, as did their approach to medicine. Outside of triage tents on the battlefield, people had few medical institutions to go to in the

---

7 Patricia A. Watson, *The Angelical Conjunction: The Preacher-Physicians of Colonial New England* (Knoxville: Univ. of Tennessee Press, 1991), 7-17.
8 Ibid.

event of an emergency. Instead, house calls were the norm. But what did that look like?

On November 23, 1801, nineteen-year-old Philip Hamilton, the son of Founding Father Alexander Hamilton, took a boat across the Hudson to Weehawken, New Jersey.[9] Equipped with a pistol, Philip prepared himself for a duel with twenty-seven-year-old lawyer, George Eacker, a vocal critic of Philip's father.[10] Initially, when the two faced each other for the duel, neither raised their weapons. Eventually though, both men aimed their pistols at one another, and Eacker fired his gun first, mortally wounding Hamilton.[11] He was rushed to a family member's home, where a doctor came to meet him and tend to his wounds. Philip Hamilton died fourteen hours later, his mother and father at his side.[12]

Apart from its historical importance, Philip Hamilton's death is also important when examining the evolution of medicine in the United States. Much like his father's death as a result of his own duel on the same dueling ground in Weehawken three years later, Philip did not die in a hospital or in triage; he died inside someone's home. The doctor came to him on a house call. Today, if someone is shot, the bystanders would either call an ambulance or acquaintances would rush the victim to the emergency room. We do not have another option when seeking professional medical attention.

---

9   "Philip Hamilton (1782-1801)," *American Experience*, Public Broadcasting Service, accessed June 2, 2020.

10   Ibid.

11   Ibid.

12   Ibid.

Outside of wilderness emergency medicine, health care today revolves around a doctor's office, urgent care, or the hospital. Currently, in 2020, the United States has over six thousand hospitals across the country in categories such as for-profit, nonprofit, community, and long-term institutions.[13] To better understand how we can improve our current health care system, we must examine how we've gone from a single doctor treating a gunshot wound in the bedroom of someone's home 220 years ago to lifesaving ambulatory services and hospital wings dedicated to certain specialties.

Without hospitals, how were doctors trained? Before hospitals and medical schools, those hoping to become physicians studied under doctors as an apprentice or, if they could afford it, would travel to Europe to attend medical school.[14] It wasn't until 1765—just a decade before America gained independence—that two Philadelphia doctors established the first medical school in the colonies.[15]

Beginning in the early 1800s—several decades following the War of Independence—physicians founded their own medical schools. However, unlike the stringent requirements for admittance that exist today, entrance into these programs was relatively easy so as to guarantee a source of income for the educators. Since these programs were in their infancy and produced less than adequate physicians, those looking

---

13   American Hospital Association, "Fast Facts on US Hospitals, 2020," Data and Insights, AHA, last modified March 2020.

14   National Institutes of Health, "200 Years of American Medicine," National Library of Medicine, NIH, accessed May, 2020.

15   Ibid.

to become truly skilled in medical practice continued to go to Europe to receive their education.[16]

Medicine was much more individualized as the time. Mothers were tasked with treating their sick children in whatever ways they could. Physicians made house calls in the event of an emergency, such as Philip Hamilton's gunshot wound, or a serious illness. It wasn't until the nineteenth century that organized medicine and medical education became more commonplace.

The United States was failing to properly educate its medical students, which contributed to the delay in a developed and organized medical system in the country. If your best and brightest minds leave to seek training elsewhere, it's almost impossible to create a stable, competitive medical education system. Human capital flight, which is also known as brain drains—"the departure of educated or professional people from one country, economic sector, or field for another usually for better pay or living conditions"—impact communities, especially rural ones, to this day.[17] The population's level of education has more often than not informed geographic mobility because an area with highly educated individuals meant more opportunities to accumulate wealth; even after the Civil War, American students went to Europe to study.

In the late 1870s, change within both the medical education system and the medical profession began to occur thanks to widespread educational reforms across the board.

---

16   Ibid.
17   Merriam-Webster, c.v. "brain drain (n.)," accessed May 29, 2020.

Both Harvard College and Johns Hopkins University developed extensive medical educational curriculums with hopes of attracting medical students to their institutions.[18] Johns Hopkins' model of a research-focused graduate curriculum, their elaborate undergraduate studies, and their development of the first residency program kickstarted unprecedented growth in medical education in the United States.[19]

We have had just over a century of development in the modern medical education system, and even less for the modern-day hospital system. Pennsylvania Hospital, the first hospital in the United States, was founded prior to the Revolution.[20] However, the country didn't see a rise in the development of hospitals around the country until the mid-nineteenth century.[21] The need for hospitals due to a growing population and the devastating toll of the Civil War illuminates the reason why new hospitals began to pop up, but these were not the hospitals we know now; these were wards to treat the sick and injured, often all in the same space. These wards were the birth of public health organizations, many of which had and continue to have a crucial part in improving health outcomes in America. They also led to the creation of the U.S. Public Health Service in 1902 that eventually led to our modern hospital system.[22]

---

18 National Institutes of Health, "200 Years of American Medicine."
19 Ibid.
20 Penn Medicine, "Pennsylvania Hospital History: Stories—Nation's First Hospital," Penn Medicine, University of Pennsylvania, accessed July 2, 2020.
21 National Institutes of Health, "200 Years of American Medicine."
22 Scott Harrah, "American Medical Milestones Since Independence in 1776," *UMHS Endeavor* (blog), St. Kitts: University of Medicine and Health Sciences, last modified July 3, 2013.

In 1751, Benjamin Franklin and Dr. Thomas Bond founded the nation's first hospital with the intent of caring "for the sick-poor and insane who were wandering the streets of Philadelphia."[23] Their mission to care for those who could not care for themselves is one of the first organized examples of public health in the United States. Interestingly, even in the mid-eighteenth century, the notion of a hospital only servicing a city and not the surrounding rural communities was a concern, as evidenced by the objections from members of the Pennsylvania Assembly who believed the hospital would only be serviceable for those who lived in Philadelphia.[24] This concern is still a pervasive one even today, especially as hospitals in rural communities close. It doesn't matter how advanced our medicine has become if countless communities do not have access to the necessary resources. That was the entire reason why Franklin and Bond founded Pennsylvania Hospital—to help people.

While it seems like Franklin and Bond had good intentions with the creation of the Pennsylvania Hospital, at the time, hospitals were places that the poor went to die rather than to be saved. During that time, the general consensus regarding poverty and illness was that disease was a result of substandard living conditions. Politicians peddled the idea that those who lived in poverty were lesser than, had lesser morals, and were at fault for their poor health. This idea, although masked as concern for other issues, is most definitely still pervasive in how we talk about health care and approach any potential reform today. This logic serves as one of the barriers to

---

23   University of Pennsylvania, "Pennsylvania Hospital History: Stories – Nation's First Hospital."

24   Ibid.

developing the proactive, integrated health care systems that America so desperately needs.

MEET THE VACCINE

Apart from the obvious, what exactly has changed in health care between 1750 and 2020? Well, fortunately, the nineteenth century ushered in a new-found approach to disease: vaccines. Vaccines are one of the best examples of preventative measures to ensure the health of a population. Although not developed until the mid-1900s, Jonas Salk's polio vaccine helped to essentially wipe the debilitating and deadly disease off the map.[25] Vaccines, new medical technology, and the growth of hospitals across the country all led to a more advanced health care system.

Prior to the twentieth century, public health was disorganized and on a "part-time basis at city, town, and village levels." [26] It's clear that medical advancements like vaccines and improvements in the technology and methods available has led to better health outcomes. However, public health holds it all together. Without systems in place for the betterment of the community that try to keep constituents safe and healthy, the whole thing falls apart. Lack of organized public health doesn't just lead to a decline in health care; it leads to a decline in society as a whole. When I am talking about public health, I don't just mean our physical bodies; I'm talking about poverty, homelessness, the environment. These

25   "Dr. Jonas Salk Announces Polio Vaccine," *History*, A&E Television Networks, accessed June 17, 2020.
26   National Institutes of Health, "200 Years of American Medicine."

are all factors that play a part in public health and impact a community's health outcomes.

With many of the advancements in medicine, much of how we approach health care requires a hospital or some sort of inpatient service, a far cry from the house call made to treat Philip Hamilton. But what if a house call system isn't a bad thing? I am not saying we should replace hospitals or doctors' offices with concierge medicine; I just believe that leveraging the technology we currently have available—such as telemedicine—to make health care more accessible could only prove beneficial. Our health care system has advanced exponentially, but we have moved away from the core of medicine: the human component.

NOT JUST OLD KNEES

In high school, I spent several summers volunteering at the local hospital. I was often assigned to the surgical ward, where I would see patients pre- and post-operation. While much of my job was helping clean or restock the rooms and transporting patients to and from their appointments in different parts of the hospital, the little time I did get to spend with the patients was time I cherished. Many of the folks I met while volunteering were older individuals who often didn't have family in the area.

I'll never forget James, an older man who was recovering from a double knee surgery (I have changed his name and the details of his surgery so as to maintain his privacy in compliance with HIPAA). I spent time transporting him between his physical therapy sessions and this recovery room. He would regale me with stories of his life, his family, and his wife. While I hold all of those memories close to my heart, the one interaction that stands out to me the most was when James first got out of surgery. His doctor came in and immediately began rattling off a list of things he could and could not do and told him what he would need to do in physical therapy in order to recover. When the doctor left, James just looked at me and smiled sadly. He said, "Not sure why the doc is so worried about me getting out of the wheelchair... I don't have anyone to walk to." Hospitals are overwhelming, scary places for most and hold bad memories for many. I understand the doctor's need to share recovery information with a patient, but the delivery was so cold and detached. When a person is lying before you, alone and in pain, you need to give them patience and humanity.

A perfect example of where the United States has gone wrong in its approach to care is mental health. I will be going more in depth into the mental health crisis that plagues America in Chapter 2, but I want to briefly touch upon it here. In the United States, one in five adults experience mental illness.[27] Twenty percent of the population is a staggering statistic and would suggest that we have the necessary comprehensive treatment in place and available. Unfortunately, that's not the reality, especially in the rural parts of the country. Lack of access to care is a public health issue that we must address and, as I have mentioned, telemedicine can improve outcomes to care by making it more

27 National Alliance on Mental Illness, "Mental Health Facts," GeneralMHFacts, NAMI, accessed June 12, 2020.

accessible (and affordable, which you can read more about in Chapters 5 and 6). In half of the countries in the world, there are fewer than four mental health workers for every hundred thousand people, a problem that rural America also faces.[28]

If the United States wants to continue to tout itself as a leader in the medical world, our health care system needs to be reevaluated. Affordability for the individual and access to care are just two—albeit major—of the countless obstacles that contribute to poorer community health, higher rates of incarceration, and over-spending. Maybe we need to bring back the concept of the house call? I don't mean having a concierge doctor rush to your bedside; I mean leveraging technology to make care more accessible. Telemedicine can serve that purpose.

In a way, telemedicine is like returning to the days of house calls. Having access to your health care provider in the palm of your hand or in the comfort of your own home feels like a call back (no pun intended) to the days of having the town doctor show up at your front door. Only this time, you don't have to actually let them in; you just need a computer. Telemedicine also provides the opportunity for privacy within the home and circumnavigates the issue of finding transportation to and from a specialist that a patient may need. Telemedicine has only just scratched the tip of the iceberg with regard to its full potential. Employing it can help emergency rooms and urgent care clinics manage overcrowding, aids

28 Blackwell, "Artificial Intelligence Meets Mental Health Therapy | Andy Blackwell | TEDxNatick - YouTube."

those without access to transportation or who are unable to take time off work to go to the doctor, and connects medical professionals to each other, thus creating a more integrated system of health care.

CHAPTER 2

CLEAN UP ON AISLE AMERICA

———

"Unfortunately, the 2020 State of Mental Health Report does not paint a rosy picture about the state of the states, or the state of the United States."

This quote comes from Nicole Fisher, a global health policy advisor on Capitol Hill, as well as founder and president of Health and Human Rights Strategies, a DC-based health care and human rights advising firm. She continues:

> Lack of resources combined with growing problem areas and illness suggest not enough is being done at the state or federal level. While there have been slight improvements in drug and alcohol use, almost all other areas of illness and access are becoming worse—for young people and adults. Perhaps this report, along with comparison to past years and additional data can shine a light on areas that are in dire need of attention, as well as show us where there have been successes to

model. But the major takeaway is that we can—and must—do better.[29]

Even before the world entered unprecedented territory from plunging into a pandemic at the start of 2020, the state of mental health in the United States was a sorry one. Mental Health America's annual *State of Mental Health in America* report found that the mental health of young people is worsening; from 2012 to 2017, there was an almost 5 percent increase in youth who reported a major depressive episode. Furthermore over 2 million kids between 12 and 17 have major depressive episodes (MDE) with severe impairment.[30] Even adults have experienced an increase in suicidal ideation (10.3 million adults have serious thoughts of suicide). [31]

The unfortunate reality of these numbers is that they predate the COVID-19 outbreak, which has only led to an increase in mental health issues; a recent study conducted by Boston University found that rates of depression have tripled in adults in the United States as a result of COVID-19.[32] MHA also found there to still be an unmet need for treatment among adults and youth.[33] "Only 28.2 percent of youth with severe MDE were receiving some consistent treatment and

29   Nicole Fisher, "State of The States: 2020 Mental Health Rankings," Forbes, last modified February 25, 2020.

30   Michele Hellebuyck, et al., *The State of Mental Health in America 2019*, Mental Health America, Inc. (Alexandria, VA, 2019).

31   Ibid.

32   Catherine K. Ettman et al., "Prevalence of Depression Symptoms in US Adults Before and During the COVID-19 Pandemic," *JAMA Network Open* 3, no. 9 (February 2020).

33   Hellebuyck, *The State of Mental Health in America 2019*.

over 10 million adults still report an unmet need for mental health care."[34]

The mental health crisis is one that affects the entire country, but we need to be particularly cognizant of how the lack of access to care, especially in the wake of the COVID-19 pandemic, is compounding illness—especially mental illness—in rural communities. Rural America has an older, sicker, and poorer population and lacks the necessary resources to manage the determinants of health.[35] Consider the toll these conditions take on a person and on a community.

Since almost 20 percent of people in the United States suffer from a mental illness and residents of rural areas are even more likely to have serious mental illness than their urban counterparts, what do we do?[36] That's one of the main questions I am looking to explore in this book. Nicole Fisher highlights the growing divide between rural and urban communities and notes the stark reality that "without a number of complementary efforts to offset the effects of population and migration shifts, the health of those in rural America will suffer."[37] Is there a one-stop-shop solution? No. Could telemedicine play into complementary efforts? Yes. I am confident it would by making care more accessible and affordable.

---

34 Ibid.
35 Nicole Fisher, "Urbanization Leaves Rural America In A Health Care Crisis," *Forbes*, last modified October 25, 2019.
36 Rural Health Information Hub, "Defining Mental Health in Rural Communities," Toolkits, RHI Hub, last modified February 12, 2019.
37 Fisher, "Urbanization Leaves Rural America In A Health Care Crisis."

A COLLEGIATE CATASTROPHE

"We are facing a national mental health crisis, and college campuses are reflecting what's going on in society at large," says Dr. Victor Schwartz, the Jed Foundation's chief medical officer.[38]

When we talk about mental health care in America, we must acknowledge the serious barriers to entry that exist. They exist both in rural areas and in metropolitan areas. They exist for poor people, for rich people, for white people, for people of color; the barriers exist for everyone. They may look different, but the stigmatization of mental illness in this country still creates a widespread, inherent barrier.

I often think about the story of Madison Holleran when it comes to mental health on college campuses. On January 17, 2014, during the winter of her freshman year at the University of Pennsylvania, where she ran track, Holleran received a phone call from her father. "Maddy, have you found a therapist down there yet?"[39] She neither had nor would find a therapist because that night, after buying gifts for her family members, 19-year-old Madison Holleran jumped off the ninth floor of a parking garage.

In an ESPN article covering Holleran's life and death, Kate Fagan dives into how on social media and to the people around her, Madison, the "star athlete, bright student,

---

38 Eden David, "Rising Suicide Rates at College Campuses Prompt Concerns over Mental Health Care," ABC News, last modified October 9, 2019.

39 Kate Fagan, "Split Image," ESPN, last modified May 7, 2015.

beloved friend" seemed to have it all together, but the Instagram photos expertly hid the reality: someone struggling.[40]

Madison's story is tragic but it's unfortunately not unique. I personally dealt with suicidal ideation in college, as did many of my peers. Everyone else seemed to have their lives together and was able to balance school, social life, sports, and family. But that wasn't usually the reality; painting a picture of the perfect life on social media was a real problem. Suicide rates on college campuses—and across all age groups—are rising at alarming rates, with suicide being the second-leading cause of death among college-aged students.[41]

These rates may be compounded on a college campus because students feel like they know everyone around them; even with the resources accessible, so many people never seek counseling because they're embarrassed. They fear running into someone they know on the way in or out of counseling, so they do not even go. I know it was an anxiety I struggled to overcome. So many people never ask for help because they don't think anyone else needs it.

I know this sounds trivial. It sounds like an easy fix, but as I've mentioned before, the idea that mental illness is an inherently negative thing and that we are weak if we show it or seek treatment for it is a pervasive cultural problem. Yes, attitudes are changing, but that doesn't erase the years of culturally stigmatizing those seeking any sort of help. It's hard to feel bad for a group of college

---

40   Ibid.
41   David, "Rising Suicide Rates at College Campuses Prompt Concerns over Mental Health Care."

students that seem to have it made. Many are wealthy or come from financially comfortable homes in safe neighborhoods, and they're getting a college education. They're pretty much going to be guaranteed a job because of their diploma. Some of them will even graduate without student debt. If there's stigma and barriers for someone like that, can you imagine what the barriers to mental health treatment in rural areas look like in poor, marginalized communities?

Stigma is an all-around societal problem, but certain groups are conditioned to place a larger emphasis on the shame surrounding mental illness. In rural areas, everyone usually knows everything about their other community members, so privacy is really difficult to come by. As a result, many people are too embarrassed to seek out help. To make matters worse, most of the time, in a small town, one's provider is someone they know. These factors combine to create a culture of reluctance to seek treatment. A benefit of telemedicine and mental health visits is that they provide an extra layer of privacy for people who have the space or a room to speak to their therapists without others around. I must recognize, however, that plenty of families or households may not have that extra layer of privacy for receiving treatment due to lack of space or other reasons.

On top of that, with smaller and more spread-out populations, rural communities lack the necessary facilities and specialists needed to provide competent care. Considering rural areas contain more racial and ethnic diversity, competency in taking into account different realities is key for "patient engagement and education and... help[s] eliminate racial and ethnic disparities in care," as called for in the American Hospital Association's Equity of Care toolkit.[42]

THE REALITY OF COSTS

Apart from competency and stigma, another barrier to care is affordability, which I discuss in more depth in Chapters 4 and 5. Rural communities have high rates of uninsured people, and there are even disparities amongst rural communities depending on Medicaid coverage. According to 2016 census data, 14 percent of the population in rural communities are uninsured compared to those rural communities that have expanded Medicare coverage so that only 8 percent of the population is uninsured.[43]

But even with insurance, mental health treatment is expensive; insurance does not often cover it, and if it does, many providers do not accept insurance. When we are talking about serious mental illness, an examination of in-patient psychiatric treatment found that the actual charge for treatment was 2.5 times higher than the cost of treatment reported by the hospitals.[44] And while the average cost of a 45- or 60-minute therapy session is $90, individuals without insurance could be paying upwards of $150 per session, with some

42 Health Research and Educational Trust, *Improving Health Equity Through Data Collection AND Use: A Guide for Hospital Leaders* (Chicago: Health Research & Educational Trust, 2011).

43 U. S. Census Bureau, "Uninsured Rates in Urban and Rural America," last modified November 6, 2018.

44 Michael Stensland et al., "An Examination of Costs, Charges, and Payments for Inpatient Psychiatric Treatment in Community Hospitals," *Psychiatric Services* 63, no. 7 (2012).

therapists costing close to $250 an hour.[45] Then, there are the other costs that one incurs when having to seek out care while living in a rural community: the time it takes to get to and from an appointment, the cost of gas, and the possibility of having to miss work in order to make an appointment. This is where telemedicine comes in. Costs incurred from the care itself as well as transportation costs and time can be cut down by accessing sessions with a provider through video calls. Telemedicine can also make up for the common problem of a lack of mental health professionals in rural areas. Telemedicine allows the patient to connect with a provider who could be located several hours away.

PRISONS AND MENTAL ILLNESS

Professionals estimate that 20 percent of people in prison suffer from a serious mental illness such as bipolar disorder, schizophrenia, or major depression.[46] Between 2000 and 2015, 50 percent of executed individuals had been diagnosed with a substance-use disorder or a mental illness.[47] Someone with a serious mental illness is not fit for prison, especially because our criminal justice system is more punitive than rehabilitative.

Asylums, which had their own host of problems, used to be much more common across the country, and if someone was mentally ill, they would be institutionalized. That's not

45 "How Much Does Therapy Cost?" Costs, Thervo, accessed August 13, 2020.

46 Treatment Advocacy Center, "Serious Mental Illness Prevalence in Jails and Prisons," Evidence & Research, TAC, accessed August 7, 2020.

47 Alisa Roth, "Prisons Are the New Asylums," *The Atlantic*, no. 4 (2018).

the case anymore. As asylums were phased out of use in the United States, more and more mentally ill individuals ended up in prisons. So, why is this happening? Are we so devoid of humanity that we expect someone suffering from paranoid schizophrenia to spend fifteen years in prison for a crime they may not even have the capacity to realize they committed? Is this the reality we want? An article in Harvard Political Review explains the effects of deinstitutionalization in the 1950s best; in response to the growth of community treatment programs and in the hope of saving money after the introduction of Medicare, state institutions began to close at a rapid rate with no viable alternatives.[48]

Prisons have become the default for so much that they are our new asylums. People who are struggling with mental illness are four and a half times more likely to end up arrested than the rest of the general population.[49] We should not be relying on a for-profit system that exploits prisoner labor to hold some of the most vulnerable populations in our country. We know that one-fifth of the prison population suffers from serious mental illness; these are not individuals with mild anxiety or depressive episodes. These are people that often need medication to function. They need a support system and a safe environment to rehabilitate. While they should be, prisons are not a safe environment to rehabilitate, unfortunately. However, that's not the reality of prisons, no matter how much we try to convince ourselves they are necessary and "teach people a lesson."

---

48 Jenna Boa, "Prisons: The New Asylums," *Harvard Political Review*, last modified March 9, 2020.

49 Ibid.

Rates of mental illness are even higher in female inmates. A study by the U.S. Bureau of Justice Statistics showed that of women incarcerated in prisons and jails, 75 percent have a mental illness.[50] Many of these cases correlate to the women being past victims of abuse, sexual or otherwise.[51]

When you pull back the curtain on the American justice system and health care in the United States, the two both fail each other. Prisons fail to rehabilitate the inmates who go back out into society and cannot function, thus creating an influx into a health care system not designed to support them. Similarly, our current health care system has not done enough to provide effective access to care—particularly for mental health—to avoid having countless mentally ill individuals end up in the prison system. It is an unfortunate cycle. Once, you go to prison, you're likely to go back.

We have to ask ourselves why some people are repeat offenders. How do we improve mental health and the resources provided in prisons? And how do we make care more accessible for the most vulnerable populations who have not yet ended up behind bars? If we can answer these questions, we have the potential to dramatically increase the productivity, safety, and health of society as well as to decrease prison populations. I recognize this is a heavy subject, but it is not one we can shy away from; we cannot talk about the healthcare system and access to healthcare without talking about our prison population. Our mental health crisis is as much an issue for our justice system as it is a public health issue.

---

50   Roth, "Prisons Are the New Asylums."
51   Boa, "Prisons: The New Asylums."

This is where you, the reader, come in. You have the power to make a difference with how you choose to spend your money and how you vote on a local and state level. Many large companies continue to use prison labor—which is modern day slavery written as a loophole into the Thirteenth Amendment—and they do not even pay taxes. Instead, consider supporting local businesses, as this not only promotes your community's local economy but also sends a message that for-profit prisons and the exploitation of inmates are unacceptable. Support the local officials in your community who want to invest in your public institutions. Supporting and funding schools, developing community centers and parks, protecting the local wildlife all contributes to healthier, safer, and happier communities. When we invest in our local institutions, we have more resources available—medical and otherwise—to support marginalized and vulnerable populations. How we spend our money and how we vote can flip the script. We have to flip it.

CHAPTER 3

WHAT THE CORONAVIRUS HELPED TO UNLOCK

———

As I sit in my studio apartment, shuddering into my blanket as the cold from the gray, rainy day seeps in, I can smell the cleaning products that graced every surface of the room this morning as I danced around with a rag and a spray bottle. Both my anxiety and boredom led to the furious deep clean of the 600 square feet I have occupied for the last eight months. With the unknown impact of the novel coronavirus (COVID-19) looming above me and everyone else, I can't help but think about how unprepared the American health care system seems to be. I am especially curious and concerned about what health outcomes will look like in the rural parts of this country that so often lack—due to no fault of their own—basic health care resources. You're probably wondering why my mind immediately goes to rural America. It's not a media talking point and as someone who lives in a city, it's not out of the ordinary to expect that my concerns would only stretch as far as the San Jose city limits. However, my experiences force me to confront the stark reality rural Americans may come to face if the spread of this virus is not contained.

It's late in the afternoon on Monday, March 16th. I'm in San Jose, and at midnight the Bay Area will be undergoing a three-week shelter in place. At this point, I've been social distancing for quite some time. My graduate school courses have gone online and my part time job at REI is on hold since they closed all their stores in response to COVID-19. So, naturally, my thoughts have been running wild with worst case scenarios. I'm young and don't have any underlying health conditions, so I'm not particularly worried about myself, but I am overwhelmed with concern for my family, friends, the elderly, the immunocompromised, the poor, the homeless… the list goes on. Unfortunately, this type of stress is nothing new for me. I often find myself overcome with what can only be described as existential dread as I dwell on the choices I have made in my life as well as on the lives of those around me. In doing so, I end up drowning in questions I will never have the answers to, and it goes on and on and on while I allow myself to spiral. As someone who lives with Generalized Anxiety Disorder, my fastidiousness permeates every aspect of my life. Those feelings are only heightened during what the World Health Organization has classified as a global pandemic.[52]

52 Bill Chappell, "Coronavirus: COVID-19 Is Now Officially A Pandemic, WHO Says," National Public Radio, last modified March 11, 2020.

The coronavirus is this mysterious, scary thing that currently occupies all twenty-four hours of the news cycle, consumes social media, and overwhelms health care systems across the globe, exposing their strengths and weaknesses. And while you may think it takes something as drastic as a pandemic to topple these seemingly indestructible institutions, the fact of the matter is the rural America's current health crisis is one that predates COVID-19. The entirety of the United States— but particularly rural America—is suffering from a health crisis in which maddening costs and a lack of access to the proper resources plague communities.

There's no question that health care in the United States is a mess. I am not talking about health insurance; I'm talking about the actual systems of care that are in place. However, health insurance and care have become synonymous. Making actual improvements to the system is almost impossible because even broaching the topic of health care breeds a partisan argument over how insurance should work. One of the reasons why health care in the United States is falling apart is because of the marriage to health insurance (see Chapter 6 for an in-depth breakdown of health insurance in the United States). So, while medical breakthroughs and technological innovations happen basically nonstop, the system, as a whole, struggles to keep up because it is caught in a game of partisan Monopoly. And there is no better example how our health care system is failing us than right now than COVID-19.

Countless rural counties in the U.S. lack trauma centers, they have a shortage of medical specialists, and the people outnumber the providers on a much larger scale than in urban areas. In emergencies, people may be hours away from the nearest medical facility that has the necessary level of care needed (see Chapter 8 for examples of this). Using data from the *Journal of Rural Health*, Dr. David Peters, a professor of rural sociology at Iowa State, broke down how rural communities and metropolitan areas are susceptible in different ways. Taking into account seven distinct factors—health compromised, nursing homes, meat processing plants, population density, diabetes risk, 65 and over population, and group quarters—semi-rural and rural communities are much more susceptible to COVID-19.[53]

The spread of COVID-19 was slow to reach rural communities, but as of early April 2020, the disease had "reached more than two-thirds of the country's rural counties."[54] Local officials and doctors alike fear the potential toll of overwhelming the already strained local health care systems, considering rural communities tend to be "older, poorer, and sicker than much of the country."[55] While governors of the states that have held out on implementing shelter-in-place orders argue that the rural nature of their states better equip them in avoiding the spread such as Governor Kristi Noem (R) of South Dakota, doctors and health experts in rural communities fear that their health care systems will become overwhelmed since they have "fewer hospital beds, ventilators and nurses to handle the onslaught."[56] So, while Governor Noem is correct in differentiating South Dakota from New

---

53 David J. Peters, "Rural America Is More Vulnerable to COVID-19 Than Cities Are, and It's Starting to Show," *The Conversation*, last modified June 19, 2020.

54 Jack Healy et al., "Coronavirus Was Slow to Spread to Rural America, Not Anymore," *New York Times*, April 8, 2020.

55 Ibid.

56 Ibid.

York, even with a smaller, more spread-out population, the effects of the virus could still devastate rural communities, considering they are behind the curve compared to urban areas.[57] In Nebraska, Kim Engle, the director of the Panhandle Public Health District, worries about how to manage a potential outbreak considering there are only thirty-one available ventilators for the almost 90,000 person population in her 15,000-square-mile district.[58]

So, while the U.S. President said that rural counties were in the clear and had the potential to open up "literally tomorrow," as he stated in mid-April, an analysis of the spread of COVID-19 in the May 2020 edition of *Time* magazine found that "the virus is only just now arriving in much of rural America. That means some of these sparsely populated areas could be letting down their guard just as the disease is about to hit."[59] When faced with the reality that rural residents are more likely to be uninsured and are less likely to receive some types of health care like tests for various chronic conditions, it forces one to pause and think about how this may reflect rural communities' response in the face of a potential spread of COVID-19.[60] If rural citizens are less likely to get tested for chronic conditions, and this behavior transfers to how people respond to the virus, the chance of rural health care systems getting overwhelmed feels more and more likely.

---

57 Ibid.
58 Vera Bergengruen, "Rural America Risks Letting Down Its Guard Just as Coronavirus Is About to Hit," *Time*, May 5, 2020.
59 Ibid.
60 Georgetown University, "Rural and Urban Health," Health Policy Institute, Georgetown University, accessed July 10, 2020.

I don't say this with the intention of being alarmist but with genuine concern. I also hope to highlight the drastic differences in preparedness and resource accessibility in rural communities compared to cities.[61] Even now, lawmakers are begging Congress for more funding for their rural towns as their populations are much more susceptible to COVID-19. Telemedicine would be useful in offloading any non-emergency issues to doctors or other specialists who may be more equipped to handle them. This is especially true in the case of treating mental illness during this pandemic. The implications of a community plagued by wide-spread anxiety and depression—a situation which may make skeptics comprehend the severity of mental illness but would only prove to be harmful overall—would only be exacerbated in rural communities that lack the proper recourses to provide mental health care for their residents. Telemedicine is in the position to help offset the system for mental health reasons or any other medical issue that doesn't require an in-person consultation.

In writing this book, I am examining how to develop a more community-based approach to health. Someone should not have to live in an urban area in order to access the care they so desperately need. One way that accessibility can be drastically improved is through the use of telemedicine. The legislation surrounding telemedicine that is currently in place in the United States is vague and in desperate need of an update.

---

61 By the time this book is published, we will have a much better understanding of how COVID-19 affected rural communities and I can only hope the impact is minimal, but I am writing about this at length because it paints a broader picture for the need to reform health care to better suit the needs of those living in more remote areas.

Many of the laws outlining how telehealth may be implemented and how insurance reimbursement works are over a decade old. Also, the online infrastructure is not adequate, either. Much of rural America suffers from a lack of internet and thus, even if local communities attempted to implement telemedicine practices, this would be a massive obstacle to navigate. In the ever-changing technological landscape, it is the job of our local, state, and federal legislators to keep up with the times. It is my dream that this book starts a dialogue about necessary policy and infrastructure changes to allow insurance companies and state and local governments to work with hospitals and health care systems to invest in and grow telemedicine practices so no city, town, or person is left behind.

WHY NOW?

When I set out to write this book, I was blissfully unaware of what 2020 would bring to both the United States and to the world. I just knew that addressing disparities in access to care and the role telemedicine could play in transforming rural health outcomes was important. But our new reality is one in which telemedicine is becoming the norm and easier to advocate for.

Fast forward to late one night in May, as I write this. People have felt the effects of COVID-19 throughout the world. The United States is just one of many countries still operating under shelter-in-place orders, depending on what state you live in. It's been over two months since self-isolating began in the Bay Area, and across the country, the reality of the virus leading to a potential mental health crisis begins to inch closer. I've lived with and have been highly functional with GAD as well as sporadic depressive episodes for most of my life, having seen several therapists at different points in time. But now, I am so overcome with anxiety brought on by the isolation and the sense of impending doom that I've finally gotten around to getting a new therapist since moving across the country to California. To be blunt, I'm not sure I would be able to make it through the rest of quarantine without at least one hospitalization due to a breakdown, without a therapist. We "meet" every Tuesday afternoon over Zoom, and it has made all the difference in maintaining my sanity.

I know that I am not alone in feeling this way. Without access to in-person mental health care due to the virus and the detrimental effects of isolation, it is no wonder our mental health is deteriorating. We currently live in a world where we are constantly bombarded with worrisome news, the unemployment rate is the highest it's been since the Great Depression, the economy is one giant question mark, and we are kept from being in the presence of the people we have come to rely on to support us. All things considered, it's no surprise that data from a Kaiser Family Foundation poll showed that "Americans increasingly are experiencing heightened feelings of anxiety, depression, and suicidal thoughts amid the coronavirus epidemic."[62] But how bad is it, really?

The Substance Abuse and Mental Health Services Administration's Disaster Distress Hotline has seen an 891 percent increase in calls in March 2020 compared to March of 2019.[63]

---

62   Ashley F. Antonelli, "Weekly Line: Covid-19 May Be Creating a Mental Health Crisis," Advisory Board, last modified April 17, 2020.

63   Ibid.

This staggering increase in call volume reflects the overall growing crisis in mental health and the need for behavioral health services that are accessible to anyone during the time of COVID-19 and beyond.

Technology the path forward for the future of health care because it has the ability to transform access to care and health outcomes. Never has this been truer than in response to the mental health crisis the United States and around the world during and in the aftermath of the coronavirus pandemic. In a TEDx talk on artificial intelligence in mental health therapy in Massachusetts, Andy Blackwell, Chief Science Officer at Ieso Digital Health—a health tech company that "uses deep learning to decode and democratize the treatment of mental health conditions"—pointed out the concerning fact that in half the countries in the world, there are fewer than four mental health workers for every 100,000 people.[64] This utter lack of mental health resources is the same stark reality for not only rural America but America as a whole, since it is estimated that close to 50 percent of the U.S. does not have an adequate number of mental health professionals to meet and fulfill the needs of patients.[65]

Due to social distancing and the inability to host in-person sessions, countless behavioral health programs are expanding their services to telemedicine platforms. Even the government is expanding Medicaid coverage for telemedicine. This is a clear solution in reducing the burden of increased mental

---

64 Blackwell, "Artificial Intelligence Meets Mental Health Therapy | Andy Blackwell | TEDxNatick - YouTube."

65 Antonelli, "Weekly Line: COVID-19 May Be Creating a Mental Health Crisis."

illness during the virus. An April 2020 paper released in the journal *Telemedicine and eHealth* explains, "Examples of and evidence to support the effectiveness of tele mental health are fairly diverse, especially in the context of depression, anxiety, and PTSD. Videoconferencing, online forums, smartphone apps, text-messaging, and e-mails have been shown to be useful communication methods for the delivery of mental health services."[66]

In response to the coronavirus pandemic, the use of telebehavioral health services in the United States has expanded. Telemedicine is now one of the main ways mental health professionals can get in touch with patients, and people can also use it to consult with primary care providers or specialists. Right in front of us, we are watching how mental health care is being forced to adapt and how telemedicine is bridging the gap for behavioral health treatments.

In response to the pandemic, we have even seen states make legislative adjustments to telemedicine regulations in order to increase reimbursement and access.[67] Chuck Ingoglia, CEO of the National Council for Behavioral Health notes, "We're seeing a lot of states respond by proposing pretty radical changes to their telehealth reimbursement policies both by increasing types of services that can be delivered by telehealth, the types of professionals that can deliver those

---

66 Xiaoyun Zhou et al., "The Role of Telehealth in Reducing the Mental Health Burden from COVID-1," *Telemedicine and e-Health* 26, no. 4 (2020).

67 Rachel Conrad et al., "Expanding Telemental Health in Response to the COVID-19 Pandemic," Psychiatric Times, last modified April 7, 2020.

services, as well as thinking very broadly about the types of technologies that can be used."[68]

Some states have even gone so far as to require private insurance to waive copayments on telemedicine services, like Governor Cuomo did when he authorized New York's Office of Mental Health Programs to waive certain telemedicine regulatory requirements in order to avoid barring access to treatment.[69] The Federal Government has even waived HIPAA-related penalties for providers using communication services such as Skype or FaceTime with a patient, in good faith.[70] Medicaid has also expanded telemedicine coverage with the 1135 waiver.[71] for specifics on the waiver and Medicaid, refer to Chapter 6.

Even the way doctors are prescribing medication is changing, as the Drug Enforcement Agency is placing a temporary lift on the Ryan Haight Act—a 2008 law that requires health care providers to conduct an in-person exam initially before a controlled substance can be prescribed electronically—and allowing doctors to prescribe medication via video call in place of an in-person consultation and evaluation.[72] This exception, which is vaguely defined to last as long

68 Sandhya Raman, "Mental Health Care Adapts to Telehealth Because of COVID-19," *Roll Call*, last modified March 19, 2020.

69 Conrad et al., "Expanding Telemental Health in Response to the COVID-19 Pandemic."

70 Ibid.

71 Centers for Medicare and Medicaid Services. "Medicare Telemedicine Health Care Provided Fact Sheet." Newsroom. Last modified March 17, 2020.

72 Amanda Enyeart et al., "DEA Changes Controlled Substances Requirements During Public Health Emergency." *National Law Review* X, no. 79 (2020).

as COVID-19 remains a public health emergency, opens the door to improved access to mental health professionals who have the ability to prescribe medication.

The reality of the long-term impacts of COVID-19 health- and economy-wise are devastating, but it has forced the United States to step into the future; so much of the legislation that currently exists regarding regulation and reimbursement for use of telemedicine is outdated, but shelter-in-place orders and social distancing have resulted in the entire country's reliance on telemedicine. The Federal Government, as well as individual states, has reshaped telemedicine legislation more within the past several months than they have in over a decade. When reckoning with a public health crisis that affects the entire country, the changes that rural America has desperately needed have come about much faster. This is a silver lining I will hold onto as we navigate life after COVID-19

, although we definitely aren't there yet, and I don't think things will ever really go back to the way they were. Hopefully, these impactful changes will prove sustainable and remain implemented permanently.

CHAPTER 4

ACCESS TO CARE

———

LACK OF RESOURCES AND NEGLECT

At 3:00 a.m. on a 30-degree night at the end of February 2016, 19-year-old Rachel called her mom from her hotel room in Roanoke, Virginia, complaining that she did not feel well. She was unable to get herself up to move around. Rachel had opted to spend the night at the hotel because upon landing at the Roanoke airport, she had not felt well enough to drive herself the hour back to school. Rachel's mom thought her daughter was suffering from a panic attack, so she called her daughter's university located in the town of Lexington, nestled in the Blue Ridge Mountains. The university dispatched Public Safety officers to pick her up and bring her back to campus. Upon their arrival to Rachel's hotel room, they had to pack up her belongings for her, as she was physically unable to do so herself. Something was clearly wrong.

Rachel fell asleep on the drive back to campus, the fatigue and chills overtaking her ability to stay awake. Public Safety brought her to the University Health Center where she slept for a while more before waking up to find what looked like pink and purple pinprick bruise marks all over her hands and feet. A lightbulb immediately went off in Rachel's head. Several years prior, when her older sister was nineteen, the same thing had happened to her before she was diagnosed with meningitis. She immediately informed the nurses at the health center about what she found on her hands and feet and her sister's medical history. Much like Rachel, they believed the bruises to be meningococcal septicemia, a symptom of meningitis where broken blood vessels resemble a rash. They called an ambulance and immediately sent her to the emergency room at Carilion Stonewall Jackson Hospital, a mere five minutes from campus.

Carilion Stonewall is a critical access hospital that sits atop a hill that looks out over the city's cemetery.[73] The ER is small; its entrance is immediately to the left of the main entrance and opens to the same waiting room. One or two women usually sit behind a window, ready to do patient intake. In Rachel's case, she was rushed straight to the back to one of the twenty-five beds the hospital houses. CSJH doesn't usually see much more than the occasional drunk college student, elderly patients, or people with chronic conditions. Lexington is home to just over 7,000 people, a number which swells to 10,000 during the school year when the two colleges within the city limits are in session. During their usual day to day, the hospital doesn't see much action. So, when Rachel came in, it was clear right from the get-go that they were not prepared to handle the situation.

---

73   Rural Health Information Hub, "Critical Access Hospitals (CAHs)," Topics, RHI Hub, last modified August 20, 2019.

When Rachel told me her story for this book, she recalls the frustration of being in the hospital for hours, knowing exactly what was wrong with her but having a doctor that "totally disregarded my sister's medical history and the fact that I quite obviously was showing signs of meningitis." Her doctor ran countless tests, ignoring Rachel and her mother's pleas that what she had was meningitis. During a phone call with Rachel's mother, the doctor tried to convince her that Rachel had some extremely rare disease that originated in Africa. However, in order to contract the disease, you must be of African descent, which Rachel is not. It's hard to know if the doctor's complete lack of professionalism was just an attitude problem or if they were completely unprepared to deal with a serious rare disease. Unfortunately, Rachel's experience only got worse before it got better.

When they finally decided to test Rachel for meningitis—a test that requires a lumbar puncture—the doctor attempted the spinal tap over and over, unsuccessfully. A lumbar puncture is invasive and uncomfortable, since they inject a needle between the bones in the lower spine.[74] After the doctor's seventh attempt, the hospital's anesthesiologist stepped in and successfully did it on his first attempt. The fact that Rachel had to endure this test so many times while she was extremely ill really speaks to the doctor's inexperience and the hospital's lack of preparedness. Once they finally got the positive test back for meningitis, it was clear Rachel had to be admitted long term, contrary to the doctor's previous argument that Rachel was well enough to go back to school.

---

74 National Health Services, "Lumbar Puncture," Conditions, NHS, last
   modified January 23, 2018.

To make matters worse, while Rachel's fever dangerously worsened, the hospital wouldn't release her until she paid her bill. Only after she paid the bill in full would they transfer her to the University of Virginia Medical Center, a little over an hour away in Charlottesville, where she would receive her treatment. Rachel's stay at UVA was the opposite of her stay at CSJH. Rachel called the facility "amazing" and said her nurses and doctors were attentive and respectful. We can see the blatantly obvious disconnect and lack of resources in rural communities from Rachel's stay in CSJH; not only was doctor unable to perform the lumbar puncture and had no bedside manner, but the hospital seemed unconcerned that making Rachel pay her bill before leaving could have been life-threatening for her.

The first time Rachel told me her story, I remember the expression on her face: disbelief, resignation, and fear, all at once. Every time I hear the story, I am both shocked and angry—shocked that a hospital could have been so neglectful and angry that those actions put my friend's life at risk. When I decided to write this book, I knew it meant finding and facing the worst of our health care system, head on. I just didn't think about how difficult confronting that reality would be.

The more I stop and think, the more Rachel's story just makes me sad. Hospitals like CSJH are not the exception; they're the rule. It's one of the reasons I am so passionate about transforming access to care—rural America shouldn't be left behind. Where you live in the United States should not dictate whether or not your entire community is able to access quality health care. I understand that having world-class hospitals in every town across the country unrealistic and not the point I am trying to make. Instead, I argue that not everything has to be done the traditional way. So much of medicine is innovative now, so why should that not be true for the way medical professionals administer treatment?

It would be short sighted of me not to address the challenges of adapting to using telemedicine, especially in the face of an unprecedented global health crisis forcing us to social distance and see our doctors over Zoom. These challenges look different for everybody. For some, accessing the internet is a barrier to care. For others, it is the challenge of seeking privacy or a safe space to be comfortable while on a call with a doctor or therapist. These are two issues that must be addressed on a broader scale.

An article in *The New Yorker* breaks down how remote therapy sessions have changed the dynamic between patient and therapist. According to psychologist and psychoanalyst Barbra Zuck Locker, "It's utterly different and exactly the same," by which she means that the dynamic has shifted due to more focused attention from the patient onto the provider than during in-person sessions.[75] While it may not strike you as a pressing matter in regards to how telemedicine can shape how we approach care, it does beg the question of how it changes the relationships between patient and provider and whether those changes are good or bad.

---

75 Adam Gopnik, "The New Theatrics of Remote Therapy," *The New Yorker*, May 25, 2020.

Rachel's experience is a symptom of a larger, more complex problem than just how rural health care lacks resources. It's true; rural America is significantly less likely to have medical specialists, mental health professionals, and other medical services available in more populous areas. However, take that issue and compound it with other disparities in care, such as the barriers women, people of color, and low-income individuals face. I am not going to spend time up on my soap box breaking down how racism is a public health crisis that informs the level of attention and care a patient receives and if their concerns are properly addressed, but I will leave you with this: Black women in America are three times more likely to die due to pregnancy-related causes compared to women of other races. Also, overall pregnancy-related deaths have increased in the United States in the past twenty-five years, with two-thirds of the deaths occurring during pregnancy or within a week of giving birth.[76] For more information on this topic, I implore you to read Dayna Bowen Matthew's book *Just Medicine: A Cure for Racial Inequality in America*.

These statistics are extremely concerning when considering we are supposed to live in one of the most advanced countries in the world. Systemic racism is a factor that cannot be ignored; doctors ignore Black women's medical complaints more often than their white counterparts, and doctors are more likely to ignore women's complaints—especially regarding pain—than men's. Take Connecticut resident Stacy Ann Walker, for example. Her doctor willfully ignored her

---

76   The Associated Press, "U.S. Pregnancy Deaths Are Up, Especially among Black Women," NBC News, AP, last modified May 9, 2019.

complaints when she was pregnant, and it eventually led to life-threatening complications for both herself and her baby.[77] I'm not sharing this information for inflammatory purposes; this context is crucial in understanding the different barriers in accessing health care.

CONNECTING FAMILIES TO WORLD CLASS HEALTH CARE, ONE CALL AT A TIME

During the summer of 2019, Sophie Wilks, a rising junior in college, was working on research with the pulmonology and psychology departments at Alfred I. duPont Hospital for Children. AI duPont, located in Wilmington, Delaware, is a children's hospital with doctors in countless specializations. Families travel from far and wide to seek treatment or consultation at the hospital.

"There's one family I'll never forget," she tells me over Face-Time. A mix of emotions cross her face. Was it fondness? Heartbreak? Sophie recounts how a single mom had one child with cystic fibrosis who was being treated at duPont, one with autism, and two others suffering from other health problems. She was a school bus driver, and with the father being out of the picture, money was tight. The mom was constantly scrambling to make enough to pay for treatments and nebulizers, and more often than not she couldn't make it to the scheduled appointments because she had to work. As Sophie tells me this story, it is evident that she was particularly struck by this situation. The reality of this single mom

---

77 Ibid.

and her four kids is a heartbreaking one that reveals cracks in the system. It also points to part of the solution: telemedicine.

The family lived outside of Philadelphia, which was over a 45-minute drive from duPont, so getting to the hospital was time consuming and taking time off wasn't really an option for the mom. If the appointment was not a glucose-level tolerance test, which is essentially just a blood draw, it would often be done using telemedicine. So, the mom was able to get on a call with her child's doctor, a nurse practitioner, or even the dietician, without missing work, driving an hour-and-a-half round trip, or sitting in the waiting room and through a long appointment. All she needed was a phone or tablet with internet access. If it weren't for telemedicine, her child may not have been able to receive the necessary treatment because the appointments would not have been accessible due to her job.

During the three months she was at duPont, Sophie worked on the qualitative portion of a mixed-methods study designed to develop sleep intervention for children with cystic fibrosis. She saw the positive effects of telemedicine in particularly during this sleep study; many people who lived in southern Delaware asked to do the study via telemedicine because they couldn't miss work, they had kids to take care of, and they just didn't have enough time.

The study centered around interviewing the children and parents about the child's sleep habits, which could take over an hour. Oftentimes, parents did not have the time or the means to take an hour to go to the hospital for an interview.

So, instead, they would do it over their lunch break or over the weekend via phone call or video call.

Sophie tells me that once the study for the intervention is complete, they're planning to carry out the rest of it through telemedicine in order to save families driving time and money from having to go back and forth. Telemedicine is going to be a legitimate part of this sleep study because if patients and their parents have to spend several hours driving and interviewing, many couldn't participate and it would prove almost useless. Telemedicine is really the only viable option in this situation.

One may ask why a single mom of four kids who lives outside of Philadelphia goes to a hospital in Delaware. The thing is, specialists for diseases like cystic fibrosis—which is not the rarest but is also not common—are not in every hospital. Furthermore, specialists for children are much more difficult to find. Not every city even has a major hospital with these kinds of specialists available, so telemedicine is crucial. When relying on doctor visits and checkups, particularly when those doctor visits are significantly more consistent than an annual physical, telemedicine is one of the only ways to allow that child to maintain a normal life rather than spending all their time traveling to and from the hospital and in appointments. That's why the use of telemedicine in the sleep study is so important; the entire point of the study is to improve the child's overall well-being. It's not just about treating cystic fibrosis—it's about giving the kid a better life overall, and telemedicine can help do that.

CHAPTER 5

SHOW ME THE MONEY

———

I'm on a call with Dr. Timothy Elliott, one of the founders of Texas A&M's Telebehavioral Health Program. Dr. Elliott has greying hair atop his mostly bald head, and a soul patch. He looks as if he was cool when he was younger, like the kind of cool you didn't appreciate until you grew up. He speaks with a distinct southern accent, his words dripping with gravitas. He's the kind of talker you could listen to forever because you know what he's saying matters. He also knows how to generate some laughs. However, what he's telling me is no laughing matter. Money in medicine never is. And unfortunately, we have to talk money if we want to talk about shaping the health care industry.

When I ask Dr. Elliott if he thinks framing the conversation of the reform and development of health care around money helps get people to take those much-needed steps forward into implementing change, his answer—a surprise to no one—is a resounding yes.

"I don't think there's any way around it. I mean people will have a certain amount of empathy, but we're limited."

Dr. Elliott then goes on to recount his own experience with an elected official who vocalized their frustrations with the fact that mental health issues were eating up the county's budget and questioning why people couldn't just read a self-help book to get better. It is clear that Dr. Elliott is still bothered by the interaction he had with the official who demonstrated a lack of empathy for those needing mental health care.

In 2013, localities spent over $20 billion on care that was uncompensated.[78] Harris County, Texas spent half a billion dollars in taxes on care because counties—more often than not—aren't reimbursed for the care they provide to the uninsured.[79] It's a sad reality, but Dr. Elliott is right; our society only has so much empathy. After a certain point, we have to talk business. And that's where Texas A&M's Telebehavioral Health Program succeeds.

As Dr. Elliot recounts the beginning days of Texas A&M's program to me, he makes sure to mention where their approach differed from what we're seeing now. Dr. Elliott noted that Dr. Jim Burdine, the other founder of the program, was in constant communication with leaders in the community who had identified this problem because of how much it was costing them. Community leaders and judges worked with the county commissioners court and the mayor. They all noticed every fiscal year they were in the red while trying to manage indigent care.

---

78 National Association of Counties, "Medicaid and Counties," *Understanding the Program and Why It Matters to Counties,* last modified January 2017.

79 Ibid.

For reference, mental illness is the costliest medical condition in the United States, with over $200 billion spent on treatment and care in 2016.[80] I am currently seeing a cognitive behavioral therapist to help manage my anxiety and depression. Although I have great insurance that covers part of my treatment even though my provider is out of network, I still pay $150 per session. Without insurance coverage, it would cost $250 per session. I'm lucky because I can afford to receive and pay for this treatment, but the cost is still there; my family can still feel it. There's good news, though. In an examination of telehealth in rural America, a National Rural Health Association policy brief found that the increase of costs to fund telemedicine is negligible and proposes that it could eventually lead to a cost decrease for health care by specialists, which would mitigate inpatient care costs associated with the lack of access to specialists.[81]

As we continue to chat, Dr. Elliott tells me something I find to be particularly poignant: "Regrettably, the correctional system is the largest single provider of mental health services in the country, and it costs local economies;" because the inmates didn't have access to mental health care before being incarcerated, the county ends up paying for it in other ways. The United States has a long history of incarcerating folks who suffer from mental illness. In a 2014 study, the Treatment Advocacy Center found that there were more than 350,000

80 Tim Flanagan, "America's Highest Healthcare Cost in 2016? Mental Health," HealthCare Recruiters International, last modified September 5, 2016.
81 Windy Alonso et al., *Telehealth in Rural America*, National Rural Health Association Policy Brief, accessed July 17, 2020.

inmates with serious mental illness in prisons and jails.[82] A report released by the Department of Justice in 2006 found that "15 percent of inmates of state prisons and 24 percent of inmates in local jails" suffered from psychosis.[83]

Dr. Elliott notes another problem: the "eating up of emergency room care [with] people who attempted suicide or ... harm to self or others." As a result of overcrowded ERs, law enforcement has to take these individuals to a hospital several hours away. Law enforcement then incurs costs because they must keep officers stationed with the person for several days while they are treated before they can be released or taken into custody. Then, the county has to pay for the costs incurred at the hospital, as well.

Dr. Burdine and Dr. Elliott collaborated with leaders in the community to find ways to provide necessary mental health services. After developing and implementing community access points where folks could receive care, they saw concrete changes in the community on both personal and governing levels. The Brazos Valley counties started meeting budgets and certain ones even started to come in under budget because they were saving so much money. Thanks to these doctors, people now had access to preventative mental health care rather than only having care after an emergency room visit or arrest.

---

82 E. Fuller Torrey et al., *The Treatment of Persons with Mental Illness in Prisons and Jails: A State Survey*, a joint report by Treatment Advocacy Center and National Sheriffs' Association, accessed May 18, 2020.

83 Ibid.

Dr. Elliott and the telebehavioral health program have proven to be extremely successful in their approach to helping the Brazos Valley communities, but the bottom line was always, "We're saving you money, and we're using what money you have prudently and efficiently."

California is seeing similar savings with the Full Service Partnerships (FSP), an integrated mental health program designed for individuals with severe mental illness.[84] The UCLA Center for Healthier Children, Families and Communities conducted a study that found that in the long run, the FSP leads to savings for the state. Reyna Bradley, the center's Chief of Research and Evaluation, argues, "If you take a severely downtrodden person, and look at the time they spend in the criminal justice system and in emergency rooms, those are significant costs to society." Specifically, the study found that "the state saved about 80 percent of its psychiatric hospitalization costs," and there was an overall 17 percent reduction in cost for California.[85] While Bradley notes that "the real good is helping these people," these savings are critical evidence for the importance of investing in the health care and well-being of our populations, if only for the sake of saving money.[86] Maybe I'm naïve, but I always thought it was abundantly clear that the return of investment—especially when that investment is the health of people in the community—was always be a positive. Even if there wasn't a financial incentive, the concept of a happier, healthier society would suggest a safer society, something we should all strive for.

---

84 David Gorn, "Saving Money, Lives with Mental Health Program," California Healthline, last modified November 20, 2012.

85 Ibid.

86 Ibid.

But unfortunately, like what Dr. Elliott said about empathy, people eventually max out their ability to care.

The most difficult part of shaking up American health care is convincing those who have the power to help lead the change that it is worth it. Since for-profit care is the name of the game, when there isn't a clear bottom line or opportunity to profit, there is also no interest. While treating mental illness would not fix all that is wrong with health care, the positives would so largely outweigh any negative—which would truly only be cost, It's almost unbelievable that the United States has not implemented any sort of system to guarantee access to mental health services; investment in society will yield a net positive outcome.

The Perry Preschool Project is the perfect example of this. The PPP was a study initially conducted in the 1960s that has since been reproduced multiple times. It found that enrolling students from disadvantaged backgrounds (the original study looked at African American children living in poverty) into a quality preschool compared to children with the same circumstances who did not attend preschool had a positive impact on the level of education and income the children achieved> Furthermore, it led to lower rates of criminal activity and bearing children out of wedlock, all of which were shown to be sustained through adulthood.[87] I'm a proponent for public preschool. The Head Start program is great, but it is not accessible everywhere nor to everyone. I think schooling should be handled more by the state than

87   Laura and John Arnold Foundation, "Evidence Summary for the Perry Preschool Project," *Social Programs That Work Review*, Social Programs That Work, accessed October 21, 2020.

the federal government. The Perry Preschool Project d(
an exemplary job of exhibiting why, but it also goes to show
how even small investments in communities and the people
that live there can prove to have drastic results. PPP, UCLA,
and Texas A&M all have something in common: they built
around the needs of the communities they were working for
and with, and they did not impose an assumed solution on
that population.

I think what California and Texas A&M have done, respec-
tively, needs to be adopted across the country and tailored to
suit the state's needs. Fortunately, this has already happened
in South Carolina; the state government tasked the Medical
University of South Carolina (MUSC) to develop a program
similar to Texas A&M's Telebehavioral Health Program to
be implemented in counties across the state. I will discuss
MUSC's approach, as well as Texas A&M's, in more depth
in Chapter 8.

Cost has to be a central point when we discuss change within
health care, but a cultural shift is necessary, too. Cost is more
than just a financial burden on people when they cannot
access care; cost is an emotional burden, too, and lack of
access takes a physical toll. I mentioned this previously, but
when I was not in therapy and COVID-19 shelter-in-place
had started, I was in what could only be considered a state
of despair. It was not good. I'm lucky, though, because I am
privileged enough to have quality health insurance and could
easily access a therapist through telemedicine. However, so
many people do not have this privilege. Even with telemedicine's expansion throughout the United States because of

COVID-19, the uninsured are still screwed. There's really no other way to put it.

SO, YOU WANT TO TALK ABOUT COST?

How much do we spend taking care of those that end up institutionalized or in prison because we don't have systems in place to take care of them beforehand? How much do we spend on handling people struggling with PTSD or dealing with trauma? We have so much more than just money to consider, such as time and real human lives. And yet, money will always outweigh everything else due to the way the United States health care system is structured. I'm sick of it. Honestly, someone reading this probably is going think, "Oh, she's just a girl. She doesn't know what she's talking about. This is some liberal young adult who is just idealizing a world that is not possible." To that, I respond that the United States is the only developed nation in the world without a public health care system. I find it ridiculous. Okay, we are a more populous nation than many others, but we also spend exorbitant amounts of money on things we don't need, like the military budget, just to name one. It is not hard to cut spending. This country preaches the ideals of being fiscally conservative, and yet, that is never the case. More often than not, the only time our government cuts spending is when it is an assistance or educational program.

We have been brainwashed to think that welfare is a scam and people are cheating the system; if we don't receive assistance, no one else should receive it, either. This line of thinking should be inherently un-American. The idea of the "welfare queen," an inherently derogatory and racist term, was concocted by President Reagan's administration in the 1970s and was solely based around the case of one woman.[88] This has fed into the narrative of people who intentionally remain unemployed in order to receive welfare, a thought process which has two flaws. First of all, in the Supplemental Nutrition Assistance Program (SNAP), more commonly known as food stamps, less than one percent of distributed benefits were proved fraudulent.[89] Also, less than two percent of unemployment insurance payments were based in fraud.[90] Secondly, the government does the math to decide the baseline amount of money needed to live, so if that number is larger than the set minimum wage a worker was making, maybe the problem is not that the unemployed person should work harder, but rather the current minimum wage is not sustainable.

So, if you want to talk about cost, we can talk about cost. However, we cannot just talk about monetary costs; there will always be more important things than money. I'm sick of politics dictating the outcome of people's lives—whether someone is going be able to live or not. Health care is a human right. You are not free if you are too scared to call an ambulance because you cannot afford it. Freedom does not exist if you refuse to go to the hospital because you don't have insurance to cover the care. It is not really a choice then, is it? The United States has a serious reckoning to

---

88 Bryce Covert, "The Myth of the Welfare Queen," *The New Republic,* July 2, 2019.

89 Simon Constable, "The Facts about Food Stamp Fraud," *Forbes,* April 4, 2018.

90 Erin Schnurer, "Just How Wrong Is Conventional Wisdom about Government Fraud?" *The Atlantic,* August 15, 2013.

with how it wants to play this out. The case against is always the same: it is too expensive and there are too many people. It will never work. Yet, nothing else has seemed to work, either. No one has bothered to try another method. So, why don't we try something else and, like I said before, let local governments dictate the stipulations? Communities know what they need best, so we cannot have blanket coverage; it needs to be more of a Medicaid structure than a Medicare structure. We must allow individual states to determine what they need specifically while having some federal guidelines.

This is especially crucial in our discussions surrounding mental health resources and coverage. We're in the middle of a pandemic, but we're about to enter a new one if these problems aren't solved. Not only are young people disproportionately affected by serious mental health issues right now, but also are veterans. Veteran's Affairs (VA) has made some serious progress with providing care to vets that can't afford it or can't access it through telemedicine, but the VA shouldn't have to do that for everyone. And even when the VA is succeeding, it still comes up short.

We also have a serious problem when prisons are our largest source of mental health treatment in the country. It tells us a lot of things. First, we have too many people in prison to begin with, which is a whole other topic that I don't have the space to broach in this book. I would recommend reading *The New Jim Crow* by Michelle Alexander if you want to a further look at the American prison system. Second, if prisons are where most people are getting treatment, that means our health care providers are failing and insurance is failing.

If the systems put in place to provide care are failing, they must be rebuilt, no question.

I have spent enough time in hospitals working with people in and around insurance; I get it. There is no simple solution. No one is saying there is. But we are never going to find a solution if we refuse to make any strides toward change. The left and right sides are both guilty of playing political games. They've used health care as a bargaining chip in their matches against each other, but they are playing with people's lives. Quite frankly, if that is what America wants to be, then it cannot tout itself as a free country nor as the most developed country in the world. We cannot claim that title while letting people die because they do not have enough money to go to the hospital, letting those who served in our military die by suicide because they do not have proper access to mental health resources, and allowing those who do not live in metropolitan areas to lack access to care.

I know I am ranting at this point, but it had to be said. We talk about health care in circles. I mentioned previously that healthcare should not be political, and we also need to draw this discussion out of politics. We must talk about it without the restrictions of what politicians want in the conversation, and doctors are doing that. Texas A&M took things into their own hands and are working with local leaders, but as I mentioned, even some of those leaders do not buy into it—they're doing it to save money. Thankfully, it has worked; with something like this, one failure is enough to convince people it will never work. Unfortunately, one success is not enough to convince people it *will* work, either. Herein lies the problem: we are so ready to say no to the idea of comprehensive integrated health care and coverage (I personally dislike the term Medicare for All because I think it is misleading as to what fully covered public health would look like and what is actually needed) that we do not even bother trying to see if it will succeed before scrapping the idea.

For the politicians reading this, if any are, maybe this will make more sense. The implementation of telemedicine, which would create more accessible, cost-effective care for those in rural communities, would guarantee you votes. Health care in rural America is one issue that both sides of the aisle have consistently failed to address. In fact, those who have developed solutions for their communities are in academia and medicine, not politics. So, pay attention to what's working, take note, and then ask the communities you represent what they need. I will gladly bet that you will have overwhelming support.

CHAPTER 6

THE CONVERSATION I'VE BEEN AVOIDING

———

"Come on, Anna! We've got to run faster. They're gaining on us," James huffed as we navigated our way through the dense brush. My little legs were carrying me as fast and far as they could, but we could hear Owen and his team gaining on us.

"I'm going as fast as I can!" I whined back, trying to keep pace with James while avoiding the branches whipping back toward me after James walked through them. I dared to glance back for a second and caught a glimpse of the others about 100 meters behind us. Then, I heard a snap and a scream. When I turned around, James lay before me, his calf impaled by branch. I'd never seen so much blood.

I don't remember much following James getting hurt, but do I vividly remember how his parents reacted. After he had been loaded into the ambulance that rushed him off to the hospital, his mom turned to her husband with what could only be described as fear in her eyes. "Call the insurance company. I don't know what we will do if they don't cover this."

I was seven years old when this happened, and while those words didn't mean much then, the weight they hold now never leaves me.

GOVERNMENT-FUNDED INSURANCE IN AMERICA

One hundred years ago, health insurance as we know it did not even exist. A century later, it is now the only way to properly access health care. We cannot talk about telemedicine or the state of health care in the United States without talking about health insurance, especially government-funded health insurance. During the summer of 1965, President Lyndon B. Johnson signed into law a bill that would eventually lead to what we now know as Medicare and Medicaid.[91] What initially started out as basic health insurance for the uninsured has developed into two distinctly different public insurance options in the United States.[92] Today, Medicare and Medicaid stand as major political talking points, with access to health care and insurance being one of the biggest debates currently occurring within local and state governments, as well as the Federal Government. Health insurance plans have become the corner stone for countless campaigns in the past ten years, which made one thing abundantly clear: politicians cannot seem to agree on an approach.

---

91 U.S. Centers for Medicare & Medicaid Services, "History," CMS, accessed October 21, 2020.

92 Ibid.

In order to better understand how we got to where we are with health insurance, we have to understand how it started. It is easy to confuse Medicaid and Medicare, as they are both government health insurance programs. While both help pay for expenses related to care, Medicaid is based on financial need and Medicare targets coverage for the elderly and disabled populations. While Medicaid is specific to each state (although there are federal requirements), it is funded jointly by the state and the Federal Government.[93] Medicare, however, is solely federally funded.[94]

Before picking apart what these services really are, I have to address the obvious. The United States is the only developed country in the modern world where health insurance—or rather lack thereof—and its costs are a barrier to accessing care. Quite frankly, it is appalling. When I set out to write this book, I made a promise to myself to be as apolitical as possible. I was so scared of presenting polarizing views that would alienate some of my audience that I avoided injecting my opinion into my writing at all. However, I have come to realize that if this book is just stating facts and not evaluating the current health care and insurance landscape, then it is not worth reading. The fact that my suggesting that access to health care should be a human right is considered political reveals both a moral and systemic failing within the United States. But more on that later.

So, what is Medicare and how has it evolved in the fifty-five years since President Johnson signed it into law? What used

---

93   Ibid.
94   Ibid.

to be just a basic health insurance plan for those who lacked coverage, Medicare has transformed over the years. For starters, more people have become eligible for Medicare. In 1972, the government expanded coverage to individuals aged sixty-five years or older and people with qualifying disabilities.[95] Those who suffer from end-stage renal disease—permanent kidney failure—are also eligible to qualify.[96] So while the United States by no means provides comprehensive coverage for all, we have added some improvements to federal protections of more vulnerable populations, which is a step in the right direction.

The *Original Medicare* consisted of two plans: Part A and Part B. Part A consisted of coverage for inpatient stays at hospitals or nursing facilities or for hospice care.[97] You can think of the services A covered as more long-term or emergency-based. Part B covered more general and outpatient use, such as coverage for doctor's visits, outpatient care, preventive services, and medical supplies.[98] Currently, Medicare consists of three main parts that cover different services. Recipients also have the option of a bundled package. The original Medicare plans A and B still exist. Today, people can also access Part D, which is coverage for prescription drugs.[99] Part D went into effect in 2006 after the signing of the Medicare Prescription Drug Improvement and Modernization Act of 2003 (MMA).[100]

---

95 Ibid.
96 Ibid.
97 U.S. Centers for Medicare & Medicaid Services, "What's Medicare?" Medicare, accessed October 21, 2020.
98 Ibid.
99 Ibid.
100 U.S. Center for Medicaid and Medicaid Services, "History."

The MMA also led to the creation of Medicare Advantage, otherwise known as Part C.[101] Medicare Advantage serves as an alternative to the original plan, as it is a bundled option that includes Part A and Part B. Oftentimes, people are able to include Part D as well.[102] Medicare Advantage is the closest this country has gotten to government-funded comprehensive health care coverage. Changing attitudes regarding health care like the increased support of Medicare for All has led to sweeping changes, the biggest of which came during President Obama's first term.

In 2010, under the Obama administration, the Affordable Care Act (ACA) went into effect, creating the Health Insurance Marketplace and largely polarizing DC politicians.[103] The implementation of the ACA allowed for the creation of one website on which individuals could apply for and enroll in private health insurance plans. Further, it allowed for the design and testing of how to more effectively deliver or pay for health care.[104] The ACA, although by no means perfect, has provided more and better insurance options and coverage for those with pre-existing conditions. In fact, from its enactment in 2010 until 2016, the number of uninsured Americans dropped by almost 8 percent. This number has hovered around ten percent since 2016, increasing minimally in 2017 and 2018.[105] If the past and current administrations have taught us anything, it is that everyone has an opinion

101 Ibid.
102 U.S. Center for Medicaid and Medicaid Services, "What's Medicare?"
103 U.S. Center for Medicaid and Medicaid Services, "History."
104 Ibid.
105 "How Many Americans Are Uninsured (2020)," *Policy Advice*, PolicyAdvice.net, last modified September 27, 2020.

on health insurance and, by and large, most Americans are not happy with theirs, whether it is due to high costs, lousy coverage, or both.

Under Johnson's administration, Medicaid also came into effect, although it looked different from what it is today. Initially, Medicaid provided insurance to people who were recipients of cash assistance.[106] Since then, coverage has expanded, just like Medicare's, and states are able to tailor the programs they offer. Both the state and Federal Government play a part in funding Medicaid services, thus informing the differences in services covered state to state. So, who is eligible for Medicaid? Low-income adults, children, women who are pregnant, the elderly, and people with disabilities are all individuals who qualify to be covered.[107] As of December 2019, almost 64 million people are enrolled in the Medicaid program.[108] With the implementation of the ACA, states gained the ability to expand coverage to all low-income individuals under the age of 65. So, while it does vary state by state, options like this shape the American health insurance landscape into one that is moving—albeit slowly— toward a Medicare-for-all type of system. To reiterate, I don't like calling a solution Medicare-for-All, nor do I think giving everyone Medicare is the solution.

So often, when insurance is discussed in political or medical circles, the discussion around coverage for children is nonexistent. Another joint government-funded program

---

106 U.S. Center for Medicaid and Medicaid Services, "History."
107 James McWhinney, "Medicare vs. Medicaid: What's the Difference?" Investopedia, Investopedia, last modified April 15, 2020.
108 Ibid.

that works in conjunction with Medicaid is the Children's Health Insurance Program (CHIP), which provides coverage to another 8 million on top of Medicaid.[109] Created in 1997, CHIP's purpose was to provide access to preventative care and health insurance coverage for children who were uninsured. Many of these children were part of families who lacked insurance and were otherwise ineligible for Medicaid. Like Medicaid, the plans vary by state, but all fifty do offer CHIP plans.[110] The fact that we live in a reality in which someone cannot qualify for one of the two government-funded health insurance programs but still be in such a tight financial situation that their children go uninsured speaks to the reality of how broken the health insurance system is in the United States.

With over 72 million Americans being covered by Medicaid and CHIP, they are the largest individual sources of health coverage in the country.[111] However, do not let these numbers fool you. Since Medicaid differs among the states, each state has their own parameters that they establish for who is eligible for Medicaid, the duration of coverage, the type of coverage, and the scope of it, all while adhering to certain federal guidelines. According to federal law, states must cover mandatory eligibility groups, of which there are dozens, but include low-income families and individuals receiving Supplemental Security Income, to name a couple.[112] States also

---

109 Ibid.

110 U.S. Center for Medicaid and Medicaid Services, "History".

111 Centers for Medicare & Medicaid Services, "Eligibility," Medicaid, accessed October 21, 2020.

112 Supplemental Security Income (SSI) is a federal program that provides cash assistance to meet basic needs for blind, elderly, and disabled

have to offer certain mandatory benefits in order to meet Federal Government standards. These benefits—a list of fifteen different services—include early screenings and diagnostics, family planning, pediatric services, physician services, and—something I think really speaks to the importance of preventative care—counseling for pregnant women that want to quit smoking.[113] These are vital services, and their existence suggests that the government, to some extent, acknowledges the importance of preventative care. Unfortunately for many, that care is not accessible.

The government offers a lot of optional benefits as well, which are provided at the discretion of the states. Some of the big ones to note are prescription drugs, clinical services, physical therapy, and respiratory care. The list goes on and on.[114] Some states even include things like dental care, prosthetics, and hospice care.[115] Currently, even though it is an optional benefit under federal law, every state provides coverage for outpatient drug prescriptions to anyone that is eligible.[116] Medicaid is so crucial because it is one of the only ways individuals who would otherwise be uninsured are able to have reasonable access to care., and it provides really critical health coverage for a large portion of the United States population. It is especially important when considering preventative care, which is a crucial investment; it is better to

individuals who lack an income; Centers for Medicare & Medicaid Services, "Eligibility."

113 Centers for Medicare & Medicaid Services, "Mandatory & Optional Medicaid Benefits," Medicaid, accessed October 21, 2020.

114 Centers for Medicare & Medicaid Services, "Prescription Drugs," Medicaid, accessed October 21, 2020.

115 Ibid.

116 Ibid.

pay a certain amount upfront than pay for more costly care down the line.

All of this is to say that health insurance has greatly evolved over the past seventy years. More people are covered—or rather—the qualifications for coverage have broadened. That being said, I cannot talk about health insurance without discussing those who lack it.

UNINSURED IN AMERICA AND THE IMPACT OF COVID-19

According to 2018 data from the U.S. Census Bureau, 27.5 million Americans do not have health insurance.[117] How is it possible for there to still be so many Americans without health insurance? The United States has morally failed, especially because most of those who do not have health insurance fall into lower income brackets. Age and race also come into play. We also see that non-Hispanic whites are at a lower risk of not having health insurance compared to people of color.

Based on a 2018 survey, 45 percent of people without insurance cited high costs as the major barrier to coverage. For individuals who do not qualify for public coverage—particularly for those in states that have less expansive Medicaid programs—if their job does not offer health insurance, getting covered can be seemingly impossible given how expensive private insurance can be. The average cost of a health

---

117 Jennifer Tolbert et al., *Key Facts About the Uninsured Population,* issue brief (Henry J. Kaiser Family Foundation, 2019).

insurance premium in the United States for one person, is $511 a month or $6,132 annually.[118] However, these numbers fluctuate by state. For example, the average cost of insurance in Wyoming is $9,191 annually, which is 50 percent greater than the national average. In contrast, Rhode Island's average cost is $3,426 annually, which is 29 percent lower than average.[119] One also has to consider the different plans that exist; someone can choose a plan with a high premium and low deductible or vice versa. Plus, many families have to pay for plans for each person in their family.

In high school, after my parents got divorced, it was just my mom and me. Since her job did not provide health insurance, she got us on a plan through COBRA. The Consolidated Omnibus Budget Reconciliation Act is a federal law that allows for an extension of an employer's health care coverage plan for employees and their family under certain circumstances that would end coverage, such as divorce, job termination, minimized hours, or layoffs. The insured must pay their premium, but COBRA allows them to pay the group rate that the employer negotiated as opposed to the individual rate. Coverage can last anywhere between 18 to 36 months.[120] Even with COBRA, my mom was paying over $1,000 a month for just the two of us. Countless Americans do not have the means to put at least $500 a month for each family member's health insurance. We must acknowledge that while these numbers are important and we need to

118 Price, Sterling, "Average Cost of Health Insurance (2020)," ValuePenguin, last modified October 12, 2020.

119 Ibid.

120 "Consolidated Omnibus Budget Reconciliation Act (COBRA)," Legal Information Institute, Cornell Law School, accessed October 21, 2020.

seriously consider what they are showing, they also do not paint the full picture of the cost of health insurance.

The impact of COVID-19 on the economy and our way of life will undoubtably lead to a drastic increase in individuals without health insurance. In the months following President Trump's response to the coronavirus, the Labor Department has reported that 42.6 million people in the United States have filed for unemployment. In theory, means the number of uninsured could more than double to 60 million people, especially since so many people's insurance is tied to their employment.[121]

We have to consider the changing job market in rural America, regardless of COVID-19. "There's just a general lack of economic opportunity or decreasing economic opportunity in rural areas, so the good jobs, so to speak, are ones that are largely defunct," Anjana Sreedhar, an administrative fellow at New York University's Langone Health and author of *Healthcare of a Thousand Slights*, tells me over the phone. "Jobs in the coal mines and the factories have largely been shuttered as we move toward clean energy, and a lot of factory jobs have been shipped overseas because of globalization, so there's that lack of economic opportunity." The binding of health insurance to work is wildly detrimental, as we are seeing its widespread effects in the era of COVID-19. Unfortunately, this especially hurts rural communities who have been losing jobs as industries relocate or shut down. Given the uncertainty of the long-term impact of COVID-19, many

---

121 Anneken Tappe, "Nearly 43 Million Americans Have Filed for Unemployment Benefits during the Pandemic," CNN. Cable News Network, last modified June 4, 2020.

more could lose jobs providing them health insurance or the means to continue paying for insurance.

It's important to note that rates of preventative care are lower for the uninsured.[122] A 2014 study found that uninsured individuals have significantly higher odds of not receiving any sort of preventative service; even with something as simple as a routine physical, only about 46 percent of those who are uninsured receive one.[123] And when considering any general measures such as a physical, flu shot, colon cancer screening, pap smear, cholesterol, blood pressure, or mammogram, almost 30 percent of uninsured folks have not received any form of preventative care compared to just the 5 percent who are privately insured and 4 percent who are publicly insured.[124] Access to care—particularly to preventative care—is crucial for the overall health of a person and for the bottom line of a community.

A lack of insurance means worse levels of access to care compared to people who are covered. In 2018, 20 percent of adults who did not have health insurance did not receive necessary medical care because of the expense.[125] In an interview with PBS in 2000 about the impact of the uninsured on the health care system, the late Dr. Ewe Reinhardt, a health economics expert and former professor of political economy at Princeton University, said "If they can afford to go to the doctor, fine. If not, they don't go." When it is serious, they will head

---

122 Tolbert et al., *Key Facts about the Uninsured Population.*
123 Lisa M. Lines et al., *Insurance Coverage and Preventative Care among Adults,* (Research Triangle Park, NC: RTI Press, 2014).
124 Ibid.
125 Tolbert et al., *Key Facts about the Uninsured Population.*

to an emergency room, since the hospital is obligated to care for them because of the "universal catastrophic insurance policy."[126]

Reinhardt suggests that this is "an extremely inefficient way to provide health care, because you usually wait until people are really sick and then you have to do all kinds of expensive things. Plus, we do know that uninsured people die earlier and die at a higher rate from the same illnesses simply because they go too late. Why do we let it go to this critical phase? Why can't we give these people an insurance policy? It might actually be cheaper."[127]

In fact, the uninsured are less likely than those with coverage to use any health services, and they actually have, on average, lower expenditures for services.[128] Due to the lack of utilization, the uninsured have "higher morbidity and mortality as a result of using fewer and less appropriate health care services."[129] Dr. Sherry Glied, the dean of New York University's Robert F. Wagner School of Public Service, said, "The people who are most at risk today are those who have no health insurance at all." Even a minor medical emergency could wipe someone out financially—a reality even for those with insurance—or could lead to a major medical issue if they

---

126 Uwe E. Reinhardt, interview by KQED, *Healthcare Crisis: Who's at Risk?*, PBS, (2000).

127 Ibid.

128 Institute of Medicine Committee on the Consequences of Uninsurance, "Spending on Health Care for Uninsured Americans: How Much, and Who Pays?" in *Hidden Costs, Values Lost: Uninsurance in America*, rvwd. by Hugh H. Tilson and Joseph P. Newhouse (Washington, DC: National Academies Press, 2003), 38.

129 Ibid.

ignore the initial warning signs.[130] The financial implications and negative health outcomes do not just affect the uninsured but can also lead to a strain on the health care system and society as a whole. I am not attempting to paint people who don't have insurance as a burden on hospitals because the opposite is true; people who need help should never be considered a burden in health care. It is rather the financial impact that is a direct result of systemic problems within our complex health insurance system that is so detrimental. It is impossible to talk about insurance and healthcare without talking about money, but the bottom line should be improving quality of lives, not profits.

Is this a global issue? Is the United States the only one with this problem? The short answer is no, but the long answer is much more complicated. The United States is essentially the only developed country in the West without socialized medicine. *Gasp*! I know the term "socialized medicine" can really set people off, but we have become too worried about the semantics. People simply cannot fathom any aspect of socialism as positive. I digress.

Dr. Reinhardt's answer to what health experts from other countries thought about our health care system will come as a shock to some but be plain as day for others; "When you go to international conferences, there's always two themes. They admire our medical clinical care, because we're advanced… and they abhor our insurance system. They call it asocial, inhumane, inegalitarian. They really think it's a horror show.

---

130 Sherry Glied, interview by KQED, *Healthcare Crisis: Who's at Risk?* PBS, (2000).

So, you have this split attitude. They come here to learn how we practice medicine, but they abhor our insurance system."[131] Asocial. Inhumane. Inegalitarian. Is that what we want our health care to be, or do we want it to be accessible and affordable for all? As Americans, we are taught to believe in the right to life for all, but our health care and insurance systems say otherwise.

With the potential for the number of uninsured people to skyrocket, now more than ever we must consider solutions. We must take into account the impact COVID-19 is having on job security, and thus the number of people who are or will become uninsured. We must consider the long-lasting effects of allowing individuals to remain without health insurance and how we approach health care in a changing landscape that will most likely incorporate social distancing much longer than we all would like.

Most importantly, we must analyze the direction we came from so that we can recognize how we need to pivot to ensure no one is left behind. No one should have to choose between paying rent and getting a routine physical just because they are not insured. We must make sure no one is uninsured.

When I asked Sreedhar about her thoughts on how we should approach health care—private versus public—she was steadfast in her answer. "Why can't we have both? It's a great idea to have government-sponsored health care for every citizen or every person who lives in America, but that's just not going to happen in [our] lifetime. I think we just have such

---

131   Uwe E. Reinhardt, *Healthcare Crisis: Who's at Risk?*

an abhorrence, culturally, in this country, to having the government provide us that level of care and provide us with that many resources. That's just kind of viewed as more of a strain on the government's money more than anything else. But I also think that entirely privatizing it is a problem… [because] they are for-profit companies that are designed to ultimately want to make a profit, right? So, that doesn't necessarily mean that their interests are aligned with that of the patient or without the employer covering the patient's health insurance."

TELEMEDICINE EXPANSION UNDER MEDICARE DUE TO COVID-19

I've discussed Medicare coverage at length, but it is crucial to discuss telemedicine coverage under Medicare and how it plays into reimbursement. Due to the impacts of the coronavirus on our day-to-day life and the shelter-in-place orders across the country, most people are unable to access the care they usually receive in the same manner. Due to these circumstances, on March 6, 2020, the Centers for Medicare & Medicaid Services (CMS) made the decision to broaden the level of telemedicine services that people enrolled in Medicare may access.[132] This decision was part of ongoing adjustments to policy regarding regulatory flexibilities.

With the telemedicine expansion under the 1135 waiver, Medicare is now able to cover the cost for telemedicine-related services within the realm of office or hospital visits across the

---

132 Centers for Medicare and Medicaid Services, "Medicare Telemedicine Health Care Provided Fact Sheet," Newsroom, last modified March 17, 2020.

entire United States, even with the virtual visit taking place in the patient's home.[133] Various providers such as doctors, clinical psychologists, licensed clinical social workers, and nurse practitioners are able to offer services to patients under this waiver.

The 1135 waiver is a drastic step in the right direction when considering the future of telemedicine. While the adjustments are being made in response to COVID-19, it is clear that establishing such systems and allowing them to succeed—even if in times of emergency—are the only ways to foster the use of telemedicine on a larger scale. It is particularly pertinent to note that before, Medicare would only pay for limited telemedicine services such as patients located in rural areas who must leave their residence to attend a clinic or hospital.[134] The quick switch and broadening of telemedicine coverage—particularly within the home—is exactly the direction we want to be heading in, and hopefully the momentum from these policy changes will allow for more growth in this area of health care across the board, not just for Medicare enrollees.

---

133 Ibid.
134 Ibid.

CHAPTER 7

THE POLITICS OF TELEMEDICINE

I get nervous when the symptoms start adding up. My body was wracked with aches and chills, the fatigue insurmountable. I'd had a sore throat the past two days and my head was in so much pain it was pulsating. My job required me to be in person, interacting with people, and while masks are mandated in Santa Clara County and I compulsively disinfected every surface around me every 30 minutes like clockwork, it was not implausible to think I could have been exposed to COVID-19.

The real question was how I could get tested. Luckily, Stanford Medical Center, urgent care centers, and Google had all established quick and easy drive-through testing. All it took was a 10-minute video chat with a doctor to confirm my symptoms, which my insurance covered because state and federal regulations surrounding telehealth reimbursement has evolved in the past months as the reality of COVID-19 settled. The changes made for Medicare and Medicaid set the precedent for private insurance, and thus, I didn't have to worry about paying for my doctor's visit or the COVID-19 test.

I'm sure I'm not alone in saying that I often find myself feeling dejected by the news that I see on TV or Twitter or read in the paper. Day after day, there is an onslaught of partisan politics. Everything feels heightened and divided, and while it could not be more pressing for the people of the United States, it often feels like a game on Capitol Hill. I am young; I had not lived through cultural or political revolutions before—or rather, none that I was consciously aware of—until summer 2020, and I was not old enough to vote until September of 2015. But there is something different about this point in time in our political landscape. I'm not pointing fingers, but it all just feels wrong. Everything feels like a game that politicians are trying to win. Democrats and Republicans act out in spite of each other in what feels like a disregard of the outcome on their constituents. To me, the current political landscape feels a lot like elementary school, when you so desperately want to be right you will do anything to make it happen. It is short sighted and clearly does not show a vision for the future.

Health care and insurance has been one of, if not the most, divisive political issues of the last decade. However, one aspect of care that has managed to draw support from Democrats and Republicans alike is telemedicine. In the previous chapter, I broke down the history of how we came to have the health insurance system that exists today, but how has that insurance and corresponding legislation dictated the role telemedicine plays in health care? Back in Chapter 1, I wrote about the birth of the house call, home-based care, and how telemedicine is an evolved version of this type of care. The idea of using the phone to limit unnecessary trips to see a doctor dates back to 1879.[135] Remote diagnostic evaluations were even imagined as early as 1925 when *Science and Invention* magazine showed a doctor using a radio to communicate with a patient and an "envisioned device" sort of like a video camera that could be used for examination.[136]

All this is to say that telemedicine is not a new idea. Its application is only becoming widespread more recently because despite bipartisan support, legislation and insurance regulations have been slow moving. One has to consider several realities about politics and our health insurance system to better understand this slow progress. First of all, we do not have an agreed upon implementation for telemedicine, since one has to consider how it would be reimbursed, if it would be at all. Everyone has a lot of questions, and while politicians on both sides of the aisle support the idea of telehealth, this is where they tend to butt heads. Second, insurance can be publicly and privately regulated, so different providers have different rules as to what qualifies as telemedicine in the first place. We must also consider that even with federally regulated public insurance, states still have room to set their own rules and decide how public insurance may approach telemedicine.

---

135 Thomas S. Nesbitt, "The Evolution of Telehealth: Where Have We Been and Where Are We Going?" in *The Role of Telehealth in an Evolving Health Care Environment: Workshop Summary*, ed. Tracy A. Lustig (Washington, DC: National Academies Press, 2012), 11.

136 Ibid.

We are currently in a time of a telemedicine boom, and fortunately, this type of care is being covered by insurance. COVID-19 effectively forced the hand of the government and private insurance companies to expand coverage for telemedicine and its reimbursement. Prior to this, the end of 2019 saw crucial telehealth progress in the form of a bipartisan, bicameral piece of legislation calling to increase the services Medicare offered relating to telehealth. Senator Brian Schatz, a Democrat from Hawaii, led this initiative in conjunction with a bill presented to the House.[137] Senator Schatz has been a leader in pushing for increased telehealth measures and has been actively working to shape the response to COVID-19.[138]

This act that Schatz introduced, known as the CONNECT (Creating Opportunities Now for Necessary and Effective Care Technologies) for Health Act, was first brought to the table in 2016 and was reworked several times before the final push. I mention this to show just how long the process can take to even get viable legislation on the table. It explains part of the reason why it has taken so long for our politics to catch up to the technology available. The lag can also be attributed to individual states, since Medicaid coverage and expansion can be regulated differently by each state. Some states like Massachusetts have been proactive in expanding the services offered; 2019 saw the introduction of five separate bills focused on expanding telehealth coverage and enhancing

---

137   Mandy Roth "New Telehealth Legislation Seeks to Expand Medicare Coverage," *HealthLeaders*, October 31, 2019.
138   "Telehealth Services," U.S. Senator Brian Schatz of Hawaii, last modified April 29, 2020.

access.[139] However, some other states have not updated their legislation, dates back to the 1970s and 1980s.

STATE LEVEL LEGISLATION AND ADVOCACY

There have also been strides made at the state level to improve telehealth access in rural communities and beyond. In Virginia, Dr. Siobhan Dunnavant, a Republican state senator and practicing OB/GYN introduced a telemedicine bill that amends the state's current plan for payment of medical services rendered through telemedicine and expands telemedicine service coverage regardless of whether a patient is accompanied by a medical provider and regardless of the originating site of care.[140] Legislation like this makes the implementation and access of care easier for both the provider and patient. Seeing these changes being made at the state level is encouraging since they are often slower to come federally, and because they can be tailored to the residents' needs in that specific state. Also, the fact that a medical provider introduced this specific bill allows for an important perspective in the writing process.

Another example of telemedicine propulsion at the state level is evidenced through Will Haskell's platform. A young Democrat in the Connecticut State Senate, Haskell was elected in 2018, and his voting record displays clear support for the advancement of telehealth services. In 2019, Senator Haskell

---

139 Nathaniel M. Lacktman, "New Massachusetts Bills Propose Telehealth Insurance Coverage, Practice Standards," *Health Care Law Today (blog)*, *Foley & Lardner LLP*, March 20, 2019.

140 V.A. General Assembly. Senate. *Telemedicine services; originating site.* SB5087. 2020 Special Session 1.

voted for a bill that expanded Connecticut's Medicaid tele-health services coverage.[141] A crucial part of his platform is his clear support for expanding telemedicine post-COVID-19, something that remains up in the air on a federal level.

Senators Dunnavant and Haskell are just two examples of the support for expanding telehealth access and coverage. This kind of commitment and energy at the state level is crucial if we want to see these kinds of changes implemented on a permanent basis at the federal level.

BROADBAND EXPANSION

While support for telehealth expansion may be robust, espe-cially for application in rural communities, implementation is much more difficult to realize. For those of us that live in metropolitan areas, it may be unconscionable to picture not having the internet at your fingertips, but millions of peo-ple do not live in this reality. According to a report by the Federal Communications Commission (FCC), 6 percent of the country does not have access "to fixed broadband ser-vice" and when looking at rural communities, this number jumps to nearly a quarter of the rural population—almost 15 million people.[142]

If we want to have legitimate conversations about expanding the implementation of telemedicine and improving access to care, particularly for rural populations, the broadband problem is one that we must address and solve. One way

---

141 "My Record," Will Haskell 2020, Will Haskell for CT, 2020.
142 Federal Communications Commission ,"Eighth Broadband Progress Report," FCC, August 23, 2012.

that politicians are trying to tackle this issue is by increasing funding for the FCC's Rural Health Care (RHC) program. A bipartisan group of Senators has called for a $2 billion investment into the RHC in the midst of the coronavirus.[143] Senator Lisa Murkowski (R-AK) said of the bill, "As we navigate the challenges of COVID-19 and ease the restrictions for telehealth use, the demand for this program will only continue to increase." She added, "This legislation is imperative to enable health care providers to increase their broadband capacity and expand their ability to provide health care to those in need." Co-sponsored by Senator Schatz, Senator John Boozman (R-AR), Senator Angus King (I-ME), Senator Ed Markey (D-MA), Senator Kevin Cramer (R-ND), Senator Dan Sullivan (R-AK), and Senator Gary Peters (D-MI), the bill proposes a host of ideas to help eliminate red tape and improve the ease in which rural health care providers can operate in order to engage in and provide telehealth services.[144]

Senator Markey of Massachusetts has long been a proponent for improving and expanding broadband connectivity in rural communities. Since the 1990s, he has been worked to improve and regulate telecommunications across the board. In a June interview on the podcast, *The Vergecast*, Markey spoke to the role he has played in improving broadband throughout his career and how COVID-19 has changed the way we consider the possibility of telemedicine. He said, "We had all the hearings about telehealth, telework, and all of that back in 1994, '95. But it's taken—in a way—the

---

143 Eric Wicklund, "Congressional Support Builds for Broadband Funding to Aid Telehealth" mHealth Intelligence, last modified May 22, 2020.
144 Ibid.

pandemic to now open people's eyes to the potential that these technologies provide for them to deal with what they felt were unavoidably pressure-packed, in-person meetings with things that can now be accomplished with Zoom." He adds, "I think it's that people still don't think as much about the broadband capacity in our country, how integral it is, how transformed our economy is, our lives are... we've just made a wholesale leap. Everyone is adjusting to it, and now let's see what the implications are. I was talking today to Harvard Pilgrim Health, to Tufts Health, to Blue Cross Blue Shield... 98 percent of their employees are still home, and that would have been unthinkable. But they're still doing all their work to make sure that these insurance companies are still providing services to people."[145]

Markey has been playing the long game with broadband and telehealth expansion, but his observation that COVID-19 has pushed up the timeline is a warning—whether he intended it that way or not—we must heed. When countless Americans still lack adequate internet access, we must make investments and changes now, or else these communities will continue to fall behind in terms of access to care, education, and a host of other necessary resources.

It is difficult to point to two, three, or even four specific politicians and say, "These are the leaders in politics when it comes to telehealth." Some names will continue to pop up, yes. Every politician has several issues they choose to focus on; that is, without a doubt, clear. With telehealth, however,

---

145 Nilay Patel and Makena Kelly, "Sen. Ed Markey on the Politics of Technology," June 16, 2020, in *The Vergecast*, podcast, MP3 audio, 57:08.

it has been particularly difficult to pinpoint those leaders because of the fact that that it ties into the healthcare debate as a whole. The healthcare debate has become so divided and so political, everything else falls to the wayside.

I do not want to be redundant when talking about telemedicine and politics, but this could be the breakthrough. Washington needs to push forward in the debate over healthcare and health insurance as a whole. If we can reach an agreement on this issue, we surely can reach agreement on everything else, or at least, a compromise. I cannot remember the last time legislation of this proportion had both bipartisan and bicameral support, at least not in the health care space. Telemedicine is the future, and even Washington, D.C. recognizes that.

I do not know who is going to lead the charge in D.C. and at the state and local levels to keep these expansions going. I have mentioned a couple of politicians who have been at the forefront, but I would not say that any of them are clear leaders in this fight. However, it is reassuring to see politicians bridging the gap to push for truly positive, necessary, and lifesaving change for their constituents and, honestly, for the United States as a whole.

CHAPTER 8

WHAT DO WE WANT THE FUTURE OF TELEMEDICINE TO LOOK LIKE?

I am in my studio apartment, sitting at the table that serves as both my work desk and my dinner table. This seat has become the space I occupy most since COVID-19 made waves across the U.S. My laptop is open, mouse hovering over the link to the Zoom call. My knees are bouncing up and down like the Energizer Bunny as I stare nervously at the screen. I check my reflection in my dark phone screen one last time to make sure I look presentable and open the link that brings me to the Zoom call.

I have always felt like meeting a therapist for the first time is a lot like a first date. As someone with anxiety and depression, I go into every session hoping my doctor likes me. When the isolation became too much and my anxiety reached an all-time high, I knew I needed to start seeing a therapist again but being new to the Bay Area posed a problem. First, I did not have a primary care provider to point me in the direction of a therapist. Second, due to COVID-19, I could not start seeing someone in person; starting to see a new therapist over Zoom in the midst of a global pandemic is not exactly easy.

Luckily, many mental health providers and behavioral therapists had already been or started providing telebehavioral health services where patients could connect with them through a secure video chat. Before the pandemic, this was beneficial for many who did not have the time to get to and from an appointment and/or were located far away from their provider. During COVID-19, this access has been crucial for the countless individuals who see a therapist or want to start seeing a therapist to do so in a safe manner. COVID-19 has completely changed how we live our lives and how we receive our care—especially care that does not need to be in person. Maybe the silver lining of it all will be that telebehavioral health will become the norm, for the sake of accessibility, ease, and opportunity.

TEXAS A&M: CREATING HEALTHIER, SAFER COMMUNITIES THROUGH TELEMEDICINE CONNECTION

When I think about the role telemedicine currently plays in health care in the United States and what I want it to look like in the future, I am hopeful. I think what is currently happening in this country and on a global level with the COVID-19 pandemic is revealing what is broken within the system. It has also forced many health care providers in this country to switch to a telehealth platform as a means of providing care to their patients. I think we are going see telehealth used on a much broader scale as a result. Now that virtual meetings of all kinds are becoming more ingrained in our lives, people are seeing the benefits, especially when talking about access for people who live in rural areas that really lack crucial health care resources.

When I think about how I want telemedicine to play a role in the future, it is impossible to not talk about integrating behavioral health into our primary care. Someone should not be going to a therapist, a primary care physician, and also maybe, on occasion, the ER but have none of those doctors communicating with each other. At the minimum, a primary care physician should be in contact with a patient's psychologist, psychiatrist, or other mental health professional. The mind and the body are not separate; your brain does not exist outside of your physical being.

Unfortunately, we think of physical ailments and mental illnesses as two different concepts, which I think is another issue of how America approaches mental health care and mental health treatment. When you start to integrate and share information about the two, it paints a much more holistic picture for the mental health professional and your primary care physician.

If your primary care physician doesn't know certain things are happening that you are relaying only to your therapist, your doctor cannot give you the treatment you deserve. And if your therapist doesn't know certain things are happening that your primary care physician is worried about, they cannot give you all-encompassing treatment.

If we integrated behavioral health with primary care, we would get much more comprehensive health care. I think telemedicine is a great way to do that, especially in rural America, because while mental health providers may not be physically located within a community, they are still accessible via phone or video call. Plus, they can still get in contact with their patient's primary care doctors. Telemedicine bridges the gap, makes communication easier, and also allows the patients more accessibility to care.

In order to talk about what the future of telehealth should look like, we must examine the leaders in the field that could act as models. I think the perfect example is Texas A&M's Telebehavioral Health Program that Dr. Jim Burdine and Dr. Timothy Elliott began in 2009 and has grown exponentially. The program covers the entire Brazos Valley, which is home to more than 350,000 people over a 5,000 square-mile area. To put that in perspective, New York City is 300 square miles and home to 8 million people. The towns in the Brazos Valley are rural, apart from College Station where Texas A&M is located, and many of the residents do not live near hospitals or mental health professionals.

Their platform works by having access points all throughout the Brazos Valley communities. So, an individual can go to one of them rather than having to travel to College Station to see a mental health provider. These local access points provide people a private place with a HIPAA compliant platform where they can talk to their therapist or another mental health professional through a video chat. They can also do so in home as well, since the platform that they use is one of the lowest broadband-required platforms; in low Wi-Fi areas like the Brazos Valley, Texas A&M's program has been able to circumvent those internet issues that you see in a lot of rural areas. However, if for some reason a patient cannot access the internet, they can speak to their provider over the phone.

The clinic truly works with the community. Texas A&M did not go in and start this clinic based on their own assumptions about what the community needed; leaders in the community came to them and said, "Hey, we have a problem: a large portion of the population needs help, and they do not have access to the care they need. As a result, we're seeing a lot of people end up in jail." Then, the counties must foot the bill and it becomes extremely expensive.

Obviously, when talking about helping people, talking about the cost is never ideal. In this situation, however, you have to talk about money because that is what really spurred the community to take action. They realized they were always in the red from paying for the abundance of prisoners and decided they needed to be proactive. So, they worked with Texas A&M to create this clinic.

Over a decade after community leaders first approached them, the clinic has expanded and has integrated with the College of Medicine as well, and psychiatrists have gotten on board. They have also integrated themselves entirely into the community; they initially started with just a few access points, but now they have points all throughout the valley.

The next step included integrating the clinic into schools and working with students. Students can have anywhere from two to four sessions with a counselor. After that, they can continue seeing that same counselor through a community access point, which allows them to avoid the issue of being referred to a different provider and having to go through the introduction process all over again. This is often where you see a large drop-off rate in seeking care because the patient has to go through the hassle of getting in contact with a new doctor and set everything up for their insurance, if that is part of the equation. In contrast, with Texas A&M, it is all the same system. Yes, the student goes from seeing the counselor in school to seeing them at a community access point, but there is no work involved with that transfer. It is significantly more streamlined.

Texas A&M has also integrated into Brazos Valley jails, which has proven to prevent costs from occurring when prisoners who serve a short sentence are released; services are accessible to them in jail and continue when they rejoin the community. Having the system completely integrated into the most crucial parts of society in the context of mental health is the way of the future.

I think schools and jails are particularly critical in the success of Texas A&M's program. In schools, they have the ability to intervene early on; teachers can talk to students and they can get the help they need. Also, the student has the ability to receive help outside of school. A person in jail can get started on their rehabilitative process and break down why they are there, how they ended up there. Then, when they are released, they still have that support. Jail is supposed to rehabilitate people so they can reenter society, not for punitive reasons; Texas A&M's program goes back to the roots of the American justice system.

Often, people and providers do not want to invest in the prison and jail population because it is not a long-term one, for the most part. With this program, however, when an individual is released from jail, they can still get help through the telebehavioral health program at the community access points.

I think that Texas A&M has created a dream scenario of what telebehavioral health should look like in rural areas, and even in society as a whole. Having these access points is key, and they have helped with mental health outcomes.

Something especially unique about Texas A&M's program that reveals the more systemic issues surrounding lack of health care in rural areas is how many of their participants are uninsured. Sixty percent of their client base is uninsured, 30 percent is on Medicare or Medicaid, and only 5 percent have private insurance, which is a reflection of the insured status of the greater Brazos Valley community and rural communities in general. Considering how much of the rural population is uninsured, if community members did not have access to this program, they would not be able to have access and care, which is troubling.

The vast majority of the rural United States does not have a system in place like the one Texas A&M and Brazos Valley have built. As the program demonstrates, investing in your community and in health care structures in the long run proves beneficial for everyone because you have a healthier population, both mentally and physically. You also have a safer population because you can work with people in the jails. As a result, you will see fewer people ending up back in prison because of the rehabilitative nature of a program like this. Finally, you will save money as a community, which local politicians should rejoice over. I mean, there is a reason that the judges and the local leaders of the Brazos Valley communities came to Texas A&M and asked to build this program: they knew it would save them money.

Do we know how to implement more programs like this one easily? No. It obviously takes a lot of work and people who were willing to listen rather than act before knowing what the problem was. So, a solution would look different for every community. I think that first, local and state governments need to identify organizations or universities that could help build similar systems.

Another leader in the field is the Medical University of South Carolina. The state of South Carolina has actually given them funding and the go ahead to develop telehealth clinics around the state. When you are seeing more of these large universities—especially the public universities working in these fields—investing in the communities that surround them, you will see a return. I think looking at Texas A&M as a leader while seeing where MUSC goes from here will result in two great examples of how we want to shape telehealth—particularly telebehavioral health for rural Americans as well as the whole country. Even in urban areas, access points could prove extremely useful, as could integrating into schools and prisons in larger and more densely populated areas.

So, what exactly is MUSC doing? In 2013, the South ⌣ lina legislature voted to fund the advancement of telehealth through MUSC.[146] Their plan for expansion was similar to what Texas A&M has implemented, but on a statewide level. Specifically, the goal is to have MUSC develop an "an open-access statewide telehealth network that will have the capabilities of connecting all providers."[147] Not to sound over the top, but this is a revolutionary call to action by the state of South Carolina. The potential that a statewide telehealth network has is unimaginable, especially for a place that is home to plenty of smaller and more rural communities.

What MUSC and the state of South Carolina have set out to do is exceptional, but even more important is the research being conducted in conjunction with the development of this network.

The research was made possible through the creation of the South Carolina Telehealth Alliance (SCTA), a collaboration between MUSC and other telehealth organizations. The SCTA was designated by the Health Resources and Services Administration (HRSA) as a National Telehealth Center of Excellence (COE) and conducts research on several realms of telehealth, including best practice and engagement. Possibly most important to the future of its implementation, they are evaluating how telemedicine impacts health care spending on both federal and local levels.[148] This is the research necessary to advance and revolutionize the use of telemedicine

---

146 "History," A Brief History of Telehealth at MUSC, Medical University of South Carolina, accessed October 21, 2020.

147 Ibid.

148 Ibid.

services across both rural and metropolitan areas of the United States.

AVERA HEALTH: HOW TELEMEDICINE IS BRIDGING THE GAP AND SAVING LIVES

In the northeastern corner of Montana that neighbors North Dakota sits the town of Westby, just 10 miles from the Canadian border.[149] With fewer than 170 residents according to the 2010 Census, there is not much more to the town than the main road running through it, the United States Post Office, and the Soo Line railroad tracks.[150] Westby is surrounded by sprawling farmland, and is so flat it feels like you can see the fields of wheat and barley rolling on forever.

On a warm evening in June 2016, several families were caravanning toward a friend's farmhouse. Amongst the swath of vehicles was an ATV carrying ten-year-old Fera Heckman, her long blonde hair catching the wind as they drove, and her friend.[151] Her mother, Melissa, drove cautiously behind, trying to keep an eagle eye on her daughter. However, several minutes into the caravan's journey, Melissa Heckman lost sight of the ATV. "I got the sense that we

---

149 "Westby, Montana," Westby, Montana (MT 59275) Profile: population, maps, real estate, averages, homes, statistics, relocation, travel, jobs, hospitals, schools, crime, moving, houses, news, sex offenders, accessed October 21, 2020.

150 "City and Town Population Totals: 2010-2019," The United States Census Bureau, United States Department of Commerce, last modified March 24, 2020.

151 Linsey Meyers, "Telemedicine—The Answer to Rural Medicine Challenges | Linsey Meyers | TEDxUSD," TEDx Talks, uploaded March 29, 2017, YouTube video, 14:23.

needed to hurry up, and another parent told me she had the same feeling."[152]

Melissa was right; by the time they caught up to the ATV, they found that it had crashed, overturning in a ditch and pinning Fera beneath it. Melissa notes, "At a typical 4-H meeting, we have no fathers along, but on this trip, we had three fathers with us." In an adrenaline-fueled panic, the fathers jumped from their trucks and raced over, surrounding the ATV. Together they lifted the several-hundred-pound vehicle off of the ten-year-old trapped underneath. Fera was breathing, but she was not moving and appeared to be unresponsive.[153]

"We were in the middle of nowhere—an hour from a hospital and twenty minutes from the highway," Melissa recalls.[154]

In the rush of dealing with the seemingly unconscious girl, they called 911 but "Melissa wanted to take her daughter to meet the ambulance at the highway to save precious [time]."[155] They could not wait, so they placed Fera in the backseat of a pickup and drove in the direction of the dispatched ambulance racing to meet them. Melissa remembers her daughter's labored breaths as she cradled her in the back of the truck. Fera was unable to speak. When they met up with the ambulance, they were still half an hour away from the hospital.

---

152 "Fera's Story: Avera ECARE Provides Immediate Intervention after ATV Turnover," Avera, Avera Health, last modified August 31, 2016.

153 Ibid.

154 Ibid.

155 Ibid.

Meanwhile, in Plentywood, Montana, nurses scrambled around Sheridan Memorial Hospital, preparing for Fera Heckman's arrival. When the ambulance transporting Fera arrived, the staff at Sheridan were prepped, but no physician was available.[156] This is common in rural areas; many hospitals do not have a doctor on site 24/7 and they often lack specialists. Telemedicine helps cover that gap until a physician is present or the patient can be transported.

In order for the hospital to get Fera the treatment she needed, they had patched a video call through to Sioux Falls over 600 miles away using Avera eCare Emergency. They connected with Dr. Brian Scow, an emergency medicine specialist. For hours, Dr. Scow guided the team at Sheridan through the care Fera needed, and they managed to re-inflate both of her lungs. Once Fera was stabilized, they were able to fly her to St. Vincent Health in Billings, Montana, where she stayed for two weeks. The ATV accident had fractured six of her ribs, broke her jaw, and fractured both of her shoulder blades, her upper right arm, and part of her spine.[157] Fera was lucky to be alive. Had it not been for the ability to patch in Dr. Scow to guide the care Fera received, she may not have seen her eleventh birthday.

Founded in 2004, Avera eCare is Avera Health's telemedicine network that offers different telemedicine capabilities—including the emergency service Fera received—to connect health care teams and professionals to meet the treatment

156 Meyers, "Telemedicine—The Answer to Rural Medicine Challenges | Linsey Meyers | TEDxUSD."
157 Ibid.

needs of patients.[158] It provides a multitude of servic₍ including behavioral health, school and correctional health, ICU, pharmacy, senior care, access to specialty clinics, and hospital services to support staff.[159] Avera Health is unique because it is an insurance company that has implemented a fully functional, integrated, and developed telemedicine system. Avera services mostly rural areas such as North and South Dakota, Nebraska, and several other less populous states, so its reliance on telemedicine is not surprising.

If one health care and insurance company is able to develop such a high-functioning telehealth network specifically designed for rural America, then we know it can be done. What is particularly encouraging about the success of Avera eCare—which is in fact the world's leading provider of telehealth—is the fact that its services have resulted in over $200 million in savings over the past decade and a half.[160] Where MUSC is conducting research on the cost efficacy of telemedicine on the state and federal level, Avera is displaying a clear ability to achieve savings using a telehealth model.

With COVID-19 forcing health professionals across the United States to use telemedicine to deliver treatment and care, we are bound to see permanent growth in the investment and development of telemedicine practices. Avera, Texas A&M, and MUSC all serve as great models to learn from and hopefully the health care industry will only improve from here.

---

158 "Avera ECARE Telemedicine," Avera eCARE Telemedicine Experts, Avera Health, accessed October 21, 2020.
159 Ibid.
160 Ibid.

CHAPTER 9

CALLING ALL GAME CHANGERS

———

As I reflect often upon my time as an intern at Ieso Digital Health, a health tech company, during the summer of 2018, I think about how those three months shaped the trajectory of my future. I completely changed my course of action academically and professionally because of my experiences that summer. I was familiar with telehealth prior to this experience, but that summer completely transformed my fundamental understanding of what telehealth was, what it can do, and what it can be for the United States' health care system. I had a much more limiting view of the capabilities of telemedicine and the use or need for it prior to my internship.

When we talk about telemedicine generally, we obviously think about the patients and the providers in terms of accessibility and cost. We think a lot about insurance and coverage that directly relates to two things: how the system itself works—so health care as a whole—and then how telehealth can be implemented and paid for—so the politics behind that insurance: the legislation. I think people in the telemedicine space talk and think a lot about the technology behind this push forward to expand telemedicine but I do not think the general public examines it as much. To better serve our communities, we have to understand what each of these platforms and products can do and offer, as well as how we can better serve different communities using a combination of different telemedicine applications.

When I think of using telemedicine in the mental health space, specifically, and what the company I interned for has been able to do in the United Kingdom by being completely integrated into the NHS, I think about the possibility of having a therapist in your pocket; a chat-based platform creates a sense of privacy because there is no need to speak out loud. Of course, a platform like this cannot serve all types of patients because some need video and audio communication. Still, the platform Ieso Digital Health has developed is wholly unique.

IESO DIGITAL HEALTH: USING ARTIFICIAL INTELLIGENCE TO POWER CHAT-BASED PSYCHOTHERAPY

The U.S. Ieso office located in Irving, Texas, has a small, open workspace and a few private rooms. Every day, they are connected to their therapist network located across the country and are in constant communication with Ieso Headquarters in Cambridge, UK. They provide online cognitive behavioral therapy through a text-based chat room that connects the member with a provider who fits into their schedule—morning, noon, or night. Ieso specifically provides a platform to therapists who treat depression, anxiety/social anxiety, obsessive compulsive disorder, phobias, post-traumatic stress disorder, stress, and sleep problems.[161]

Ieso's approach to therapy is what sets it apart; "The company has developed its own ability to capture data, analyze it, and use it to improve behavioral health outcomes."[162] Ieso leverages the data it collects and utilizes artificial intelligence to measure the effectiveness of the treatment provided and develop predictive diagnostics based on data patterns. Specifically, the artificial intelligence uses the data to develop "predictions of a patient's presenting condition, severity of presentation, and likelihood of completing a full course of therapy."[163] These tools greatly assist care providers in determining their course of action and what they need to specifically focus on in terms of patient therapy.

Ieso's use of artificial intelligence does not usurp or replace the work of the mental health care professionals; rather, it aids them and informs the treatment they provide so they can be both accurate and efficient. This kind of technology is game changing when we consider the practical applications of providing medical professionals with important patient information in a much timelier manner than would have taken them to glean through multiple sessions.

161 "Types of Mental Health Problems We Treat: Ieso Digital Health," Ieso, Ieso Digital Health, accessed October 21, 2020.

162 Kerry Curry, "The Doctor Will Text You Now," *D CEO,* March, 2018.

163 "AI-Enabled Mental Health Treatment Platform Goes Live: Ieso Digital Health," Ieso, Ieso Digital Health, accessed October 21, 2020.

AMWELL: LEVERAGING AUDIO-VISUAL APPLICATIONS TO CONNECT DOCTORS AND PATIENTS IN REAL TIME

Amwell, formerly known as American Well, is probably the most well-known telemedicine platform and company in the United States. Amwell developed their video conferencing platform and offers it through a subscription service for health care providers to use to connect with patients. Currently, the company provides telemedicine access through health care plans to over 150 million individuals, and they are partnered with over 240 health systems such as the Cleveland Clinic and over 55 health plans such as UnitedHealthcare.[164] If Amwell sounds familiar, that is because they supply the platform that Avera Health uses. In the world of telemedicine, Amwell is ubiquitous. What makes its platform special? Why are so many insurance and health care providers subscribing to their services? It is a "private, secure, HIPAA-compliant tool that allows you to safely and confidentially consult with a doctor online."[165] However, Amwell's real trick is its accessibility.

Amwell provides on-demand care; it is not appointment-based. This structure fills in the gaps between regularly scheduled care and emergency visits. It is both convenient for the patient and provider, through the ease of the platform, and it supports an often-overrun emergency system by redirecting someone who may have shown up to the ER with their concerns to accessing professional care in their own home. It is also accessible in its pricing; where an emergency room or doctor's visit for something even inconsequential could

---

164 "About Amwell," Amwell, American Well, accessed October 21, 2020.
165 "Is My Online Doctor Visit Private and Secure?" Amwell, American Well, accessed October 21, 2020.

cost hundreds or thousands of dollars, an Amwell visit costs $79.[166] The ER is often where people go in times of medical uncertainty, and the average cost per ER visit skyrocketed 176 percent from 2008 to 2017. Paying for an Amwell visit instead of an average of $1,389 could be the difference between making rent or putting food on the table.[167] This cost differential makes Amwell exponentially more accessible for people, and when you factor in the efficiency of not having to travel to the hospital or doctor's office, its benefits really add up.

DOCTOR ANYWHERE: PERSONAL AND CORPORATE HEALTH CARE IN YOUR HAND

Singapore-based telehealth startup, Doctor Anywhere, came onto the scene in 2015. Inspired by groundbreaking startups in the sector, founder Wai Mun Lim launched the company that is now a telehealth leader in Singapore and handles both personal- and corporate-level health care.[168] Since COVID-19 took hold and Singapore went into what could only be considered a nationwide lockdown save for essential services, Doctor Anywhere has seen tremendous growth. Having their feet in both personal health care and corporate-level care has proven fruitful and has gained them roughly nine times more patients than they had before.[169]

---

166 "How Much Does an Online Doctor Visit on Amwell Cost?" Amwell, American Well, accessed October 21, 2020.

167 Kenneth Alltucker, "USA Today: 'Really Astonishing': Average Cost of Hospital ER Visit Surges 176% in a Decade, Report Says," HCCI, Health Care Cost Institute, last modified June 4, 2019.

168 Fariza Salleh, "Singapore Telemedicine Startup Doctor Anywhere Thrives as Virtual Healthcare Becomes the New Normal," *Business Insider*, Insider Inc., last modified September 30, 2020.

169 Ibid.

The ability to fill prescriptions and skip having to wait in the line or pick up medications in person has drawn many users to the platform. One such user, 60-year-old Andy Ng, says, "On some mornings, the queues can stretch all the way to the next two shop units. I don't want to take the risk, and I certainly don't want to wait that long just to get my daily diabetes meds."[170] Doctor Anywhere is a great model for how telemedicine can save time both during and post pandemic so patients can quickly check in with a doctor and/or get their prescriptions filled.

A CALL TO ACTION

Admittedly, telemedicine cannot fix everything. It certainly will not solve all of the health care problems in the United States, but we live in a time where leveraging telemedicine is poised to transform access to all kinds of care in rural communities and beyond.

I leave you with this: think about what you want the world you live in to look like. Think about what kind of community you want to live in. Do you want your neighbors and friends to not seek treatment because they cannot afford it or do not have the time or means of transportation to go to an appointment? Do you want your family member to forgo seeing a therapist because she works sixty hours a week and none of the in-person providers work on weekends?

If you answered negatively to any of these questions but want to know what *you* can do to make care more accessible and

---

170 Ibid.

telemedicine more available, look no further. We can all encourage our elected officials to support telemedicine's expansion, utilize the telemedicine services already at your disposal, and spread the word. Talk about telemedicine with your family, friends, and colleagues. Share this book or share articles with those you think may be interested. COVID-19 brought telemedicine into the public conversation, but it is going to take a lot more than that for it to endure. Fortunately, even one conversation can lead to change.

ACKNOWLEDGEMENTS

————

First and foremost, I want to thank my family: Papa, Mom, Lauren, Pierre, Cata, Nico, Peter, Gui, Alex, Izzi, Louis, Diane, Mimi, Grand, Teta, and Jeddo. Thank you for encouraging me throughout this process even though you have firsthand experience of my terrible storytelling and ridiculous one woman shows.

Thank you to my friends who have supported me throughout this process. I especially thank Bobby Zipp and Harman Sidhu for putting up with me (and living with me) during the writing process. Vibha, I am so thankful I met you when I moved to California. Thank you for all the adventures we have had and the many more to come. Gabriella and Peyton, thank you for the endless analyses of Taylor Swift songs and for letting me talk about anything.

To Dylann, meatball, and pickle, thank you for all the life chats. To my App Trail Leader for life, Bishop: I would not want to spend a week in the woods with anyone else. Grace, Haille, Jocelyn, and Phoebe, thank you for your enduring friendship. Thank you, Sadie, for all the songs and playlists you sent my way. They got me through countless sleepless nights of writing.

Thank you to my high school friends Chad Novek and Liam Tracey and my college friends Mary Page Welch, Wilson Miller, Caitlin Reardon, Ben Schaeffer, Camilla Higgins, Rachel Reibach, Izzy Ryan, and Coleman Martinson. Thank you to my grad school classmates Vy Thai, Wei Nein Chen, Zoe Ding, Jeff Xi, and Zhangzhang Li.

A huge thank you to everyone I interviewed. This book came to life because of you. Thank you for the stories you share and the work that you do.

A special thank you to all of my backers throughout this process: Lesley King, Paula Kiami, Randy Karlson, Evan Cifor, Solange Johnston, Eddy Aoun, Nicholas D'Souza, Shoba Dasari, Hunter Yates, Philippe Asseily, Cynthia DeRiemer, Caroline Guertin-Villemure, Tanajia Moye-Green, Meesh Mounsdon, Rhonda Doak, Andrea Powell, and Becca Astor.

And finally, a massive thank you to New Degree Press, especially to Eric Koester, Brian Bies, Christy Mossburg, and Jacqueline Diaz-Mewis.

APPENDIX

———

INTRODUCTION

Blackwell, Andy. "Artificial Intelligence Meets Mental Health Therapy | Andy Blackwell | TEDxNatick - YouTube." TEDx Talks. Uploaded March 11, 2020. YouTube video, 18:45. https://www.youtube.com/watch?v=ZkTvw3usMw4.

Centers for Disease Control and Prevention. "Telehealth in Rural Communities." National Center for Chronic Disease Prevention and Health Promotion. Last modified August 18, 2020. https://www.cdc.gov/chronicdisease/resources/publications/factsheets/telehealth-in-rural-communities.htm.

National Institute of Mental Health. "Mental Health and Rural America: Challenges and Opportunities." NIMH. Last modified May 28, 2018. https://www.nimh.nih.gov/news/media/2018/mental-health-and-rural-america-challenges-and-opportunities.shtml.

National Institute of Mental Health. "Mental Illness." NIMH. Last modified February, 2019. https://www.nimh.nih.gov/health/statistics/mental-illness.shtml.

Office of the National Coordinator for Health Information Technology. "Telemedicine and Telehealth." Health Information Technology. Last modified September 24, 2020. https://www.healthit.gov/topic/health-it-health-care-settings/telemedicine-and-telehealth.

CHAPTER 1

A&E Television Networks. "Dr. Jonas Salk Announces Polio Vaccine." *History*. Accessed June 17, 2020. https://www.history.com/this-day-in-history/salk-announces-polio-vaccine.

American Hospital Association. "Fast Facts on U.S. Hospitals, 2020." Data and Insights. Last modified March, 2020. https://www.aha.org/statistics/fast-facts-us-hospitals.

Blackwell, Andy. "Artificial Intelligence Meets Mental Health Therapy | Andy Blackwell | TEDxNatick - YouTube." TEDx Talks. Uploaded March 11, 2020. YouTube video, 18:45. https://www.youtube.com/watch?v=ZkTvw3usMw4.

Harrah, Scott. "American Medical Milestones Since Independence in 1776." *UMHS Endeavor* (blog). St. Kitts: University of Medicine and Health Sciences, last modified July 3, 2013. https://www.umhs-sk.org/blog/american-medical-milestones-since-1776.

Merriam-Webster. s.v. "brain drain (n.)." Dictionary. Accessed May 29, 2020. https://www.merriam-webster.com/dictionary/ brain%20drain.

National Alliance on Mental Illness. "Mental Health Facts." GeneralMHFacts. Accessed June 12, 2020. https://www.nami.org/ nami/media/nami-media/infographics/generalmhfacts.pdf.

National Institutes of Health. "200 Years of American Medicine." National Library of Medicine. Accessed May 7, 2020. https:// www.nlm.nih.gov/hmd/pdf/200years.pdf.

"Philip Hamilton (1782-1801)." *American Experience.* Public Broadcasting Service. Accessed June 2, 2020. https://www.pbs.org/ wgbh/americanexperience/features/hamilton-philip-hamilton-1782-1801/.

University of Pennsylvania. "Pennsylvania Hospital History: Stories—Nation's First Hospital." Penn Medicine. Accessed July 2, 2020. https://www.uphs.upenn.edu/paharc/features/creation. html.

Watson, Patricia A. *The Angelical Conjunction: The Preacher-Physicians of Colonial New England.* Knoxville: University of Tennessee Press, 1991.

CHAPTER 2

Boa, Jenna. "Prisons: The New Asylums." *Harvard Political Review.* Last modified March 9, 2020. https://harvardpolitics.com/prisons-the-new-asylums/.

David, Eden. "Rising Suicide Rates at College Campuses Prompt Concerns over Mental Health Care." *ABC News.* Last modified October 9, 2019. https://abcnews.go.com/Health/rising-suicide-rates-college-campuses-prompt-concerns-mental/story?id=66126446.

Ettman, Catherine K., Salma M. Abdalla, Gregory H. Cohen, Laura Sampson, Patrick M. Vivier, and Sandro Galea. "Prevalence of Depression Symptoms in US Adults Before and During the COVID-19 Pandemic." *JAMA Network Open* 3, no. 9 (2020). https://doi.org/10.1001/jamanetworkopen.2020.19686.

Fagan, Kate. "Split Image." *ESPN.* Last modified May 7, 2015. http://www.espn.com/espn/feature/story/_/id/12833146/instagram-account-university-pennsylvania-runner-showed-only-part-story.

Fisher, Nicole. "State of The States: 2020 Mental Health Rankings." *Forbes*, February 25, 2020. https://www.forbes.com/sites/nicolefisher/2020/02/25/state-of-the-states-2020-mental-health-rankings/#7830afbc5ae3.

Fisher, Nicole. "Urbanization Leaves Rural America in a Health Care Crisis." *Forbes*, October 25, 2019. https://www.forbes.com/sites/nicolefisher/2019/10/25/urbanization-leaves-rural-america-in-a-health-care-crisis/#60e30e5e1b2a.

Health Research and Educational Trust. *Improving Health Equity Through Data Collection AND Use: A Guide for Hospital Leaders.* Chicago: Health Research & Educational Trust, 2011. Accessed June 11, 2020. http://www.hpoe.org/Reports-HPOE/equity-of-care-toolkit.pdf.

Hellebuyck, Michele, Madeline Halpern, Theresa Nguyen, and Danielle Fritze. *The State of Mental Health in America 2019.* Alexandria, VA: Mental Health America, Inc., 2019. Accessed June 5, 2020. https://mhanational.org/sites/default/files/2019-09/2019%20MH%20in%20America%20Final.pdf.

Roth, Alisa. "Prisons Are the New Asylums." *The Atlantic*, no. 4 (2018). https://www.theatlantic.com/magazine/archive/2018/04/very-short-book-excerpt-prisoners-or-patients/554093/.

Rural Health Information Hub. "Defining Mental Health in Rural Communities." RHI Hub. Toolkits. Last modified February 12, 2019. https://www.ruralhealthinfo.org/toolkits/mental-health/1/definition#:~:text=Mental%20health%20conditions%20are%20prevalent,experience%20a%20serious%20mental%20illness.

Stensland, Michael, Peter R. Watson, and Kyle L. Grazier. "An Examination of Costs, Charges, and Payments for Inpatient Psychiatric Treatment in Community Hospitals." *Psychiatric Services* 63, no. 7 (2012). https://doi.org/10.1176/appi.ps.201100402.

Thervo. "How Much Does Therapy Cost?" Costs. Accessed August 13, 2020. https://thervo.com/costs/how-much-does-therapy-cost.

Treatment Advocacy Center. "Serious Mental Illness Prevalence in Jails and Prisons." Evidence & Research. Accessed August 7, 2020. https://www.treatmentadvocacycenter.org/evidence-and-research/learn-more-about/3695.

U.S. Census Bureau. "Uninsured Rates in Urban and Rural America." Last modified November 6, 2018. https://www.census.gov/library/visualizations/interactive/rural-urban-uninsured.html.

CHAPTER 3

Antonelli, Ashley F. "Weekly Line: COVID-19 May Be Creating a Mental Health Crisis." Advisory Board. Last modified April 17, 2020. https://www.advisory.com/daily-briefing/2020/04/17/mental-health.

Bergengruen, Vera. "Rural America Risks Letting Down Its Guard Just as Coronavirus Is About to Hit." *Time*, May 5, 2020. https://time.com/5831319/coronavirus-rural-america/.

Blackwell, Andy. "Artificial Intelligence Meets Mental Health Therapy | Andy Blackwell | TEDxNatick - YouTube." TEDx Talks. Uploaded March 11, 2020. YouTube video, 18:45. https://www.youtube.com/watch?v=ZkTvw3usMw4.

Centers for Medicare and Medicaid Services. "Medicare Telemedicine Health Care Provided Fact Sheet." Newsroom. Last modified March 17, 2020. https://www.cms.gov/newsroom/factsheets/medicare-telemedicine-health-care-provider-fact-sheet.

Chappell, Bill. "Coronavirus: COVID-19 Is Now Officially A Pandemic, WHO Says." National Public Radio. Last modified March 11, 2020. https://www.npr.org/sections/goatsandsoda/2020/03/11/814474930/coronavirus-covid-19-is-now-officially-a-pandemic-who-says.

Conrad, Rachel, Harika Rayala, Rebekah Diamond, Bianca Busch, and Nicole Kramer. "Expanding Telemental Health in Response to the COVID-19 Pandemic." *Psychiatric Times*, April 7, 2020. https://www.psychiatrictimes.com/view/expanding-telemental-health-response-covid-19-pandemic.

Enyeart, Amanda, Marshall E. Jackson, and Lisa Schmitz Mazur. "DEA Changes Controlled Substances Requirements During Public Health Emergency." *National Law Review* X, no. 79 (2020). https://www.natlawreview.com/article/dea-person-visit-not-required-controlled-substances-prescription-during-public.

Georgetown University. "Rural and Urban Health." Health Policy Institute. Accessed July 10, 2020. https://hpi.georgetown.edu/rural/.

Healy, Jack, Sabrina Tavernise, Robert Gebeloff, and Weiyi Cai. "Coronavirus Was Slow to Spread to Rural America, Not Anymore." *New York Times*, April 8, 2020. https://www.nytimes.com/interactive/2020/04/08/us/coronavirus-rural-america-cases.html.

Peters, David J. "Rural America Is More Vulnerable to COVID-19 Than Cities Are, and It's Starting to Show." *The Conversation*. Last modified June 19, 2020. https://theconversation.com/rural-america-is-more-vulnerable-to-covid-19-than-cities-are-and-its-starting-to-show-140532.

Raman, Sandhya. "Mental Health Care Adapts to Telehealth Because of COVID-19." *Roll Call*. Last modified March 19,

2020. https://www.rollcall.com/2020/03/19/mental-health-care-adapts-to-telehealth-due-to-covid-19/.

Zhou, Xiaoyun, Centaine L. Snoswell, Louise E. Harding, Matthew Bambling, Sisira Edirippulige, Xuejun Bai, and Anthony C. Smith. "The Role of Telehealth in Reducing the Mental Health Burden from COVID-19." *Telemedicine and e-Health* 26, no. 4 (2020). https://www.liebertpub.com/doi/pdf/10.1089/tmj.2020.0068

CHAPTER 4

The Associated Press. "US Pregnancy Deaths Are Up, Especially among Black Women." NBC News. Last modified May 9, 2019. https://www.nbcnews.com/news/nbcblk/us-pregnancy-deaths-are-especially-among-black-women-n1003806.

Gopnik, Adam. "The New Theatrics of Remote Therapy." *The New Yorker,* May 25, 2020. https://www.newyorker.com/magazine/2020/06/01/the-new-theatrics-of-remote-therapy-?utm_campaign=falcon&utm_medium=social&utm_social-type=owned&utm_source=twitter&utm_brand=tny&mbid=social_twitter.

National Health Services. "Lumbar Puncture." Conditions. Last modified January 23, 2018. https://www.nhs.uk/conditions/lumbar-puncture/.

Rural Health Information Hub. "Critical Access Hospitals (CAHs)." Topics. Last modified August 20, 2019. https://www.rural-healthinfo.org/topics/critical-access-hospitals.

CHAPTER 5

Alonso, Windy, Elizabeth Crouch, and Nicol Thorell. *Telehealth in Rural America*. National Rural Health Association Policy Brief. Accessed July 17, 2020. https://www.ruralhealthweb.org/NRHA/media/Emerge_NRHA/Advocacy/Policy%20documents/2019-NRHA-Policy-Paper-Telehealth-in-Rural-America.pdf.

Constable, Simon. "The Facts About Food Stamp Fraud." *Forbes*, April 4, 2018. https://www.forbes.com/sites/simonconstable/2018/04/04/the-facts-about-food-stamp-fraud/#300f43f88061

Covert, Bryce. "The Myth of the Welfare Queen." *The New Republic*, July 2, 2019. https://newrepublic.com/article/154404/myth-welfare-queen.

Flanagan, Tim. "America's Highest Healthcare Cost in 2016? Mental Health." HealthCare Recruiters International. Last modified September 5, 2016. https://hcrnetwork.com/americas-highest-healthcare-cost-2016-mental-health/.

Gorn, David. "Saving Money, Lives with Mental Health Program." California Healthline. Last modified November 20, 2012. https://californiahealthline.org/news/study-mental-health-program-saves-money/.

Laura and John Arnold Foundation. "Evidence Summary for the Perry Preschool Project." *Social Programs That Work Review*. Social Programs That Work. Accessed October 21, 2020. https://evidencebasedprograms.org/document/perry-preschool-project-evidence-summary/#:~:text=The%20Perry%20Pre-school%20Project%2C%20carried,3%20and%204)%3B%20the.

National Association of Counties. "Medicaid and Counties." *Understanding the Program and Why It Matters to Counties.* Last modified January 2017. https://www.naco.org/sites/default/files/documents/NACo-Medicaid-Presentation-updated%20 1.26.17.pdf.

Schnurer, Erin. "Just How Wrong is Conventional Wisdom About Government Fraud?" *The Atlantic,* August 15, 2013. https://www.theatlantic.com/politics/archive/2013/08/just-how-wrong-is-conventional-wisdom-about-government-fraud/278690/.

Torrey, E. Fuller, Mary T. Sdanowicz, Aaron D. Kennard, H. Richard Lamb, Donald F. Eslinger, Michael C. Biasotti, and Doris A. Fuller. *The Treatment of Persons with Mental Illness in Prisons and Jails: A State Survey.* A Joint Report by Treatment Advocacy Center and National Sheriffs' Association. Accessed May 18, 2020. https://www.treatmentadvocacycenter.org/storage/documents/treatment-behind-bars/treatment-behind-bars.pdf.

CHAPTER 6

Centers for Medicare & Medicaid Services. "Eligibility." Medicaid. Accessed October 21, 2020. https://www.medicaid.gov/medicaid/eligibility/index.html.

Centers for Medicare & Medicaid Services. "Mandatory & Optional Medicaid Benefits." Medicaid. Accessed October 21, 2020. https://www.medicaid.gov/medicaid/benefits/mandatory-optional-medicaid-benefits/index.html.

Centers for Medicare and Medicaid Services. "Medicare Telemedicine Health Care Provided Fact Sheet." Newsroom. Last modified March 17, 2020. https://www.cms.gov/newsroom/factsheets/medicare-telemedicine-health-care-provider-fact-sheet.

Centers for Medicare & Medicaid Services. "Prescription Drugs." Medicaid. Accessed October 21, 2020. https://www.medicaid.gov/medicaid/prescription-drugs/index.html.

"Consolidated Omnibus Budget Reconciliation Act (COBRA)." Legal Information Institute. Cornell Law School. Accessed October 21, 2020. https://www.law.cornell.edu/wex/consolidated_omnibus_budget_reconciliation_act_(cobra).

"How Many Americans Are Uninsured (2020)." PolicyAdvice. PolicyAdvice.net. Last modified September 27, 2020. https://policyadvice.net/health-insurance/insights/how-many-americans-are-uninsured/.

Institute of Medicine Committee on the Consequences of Uninsurance. "Spending on Health Care for Uninsured Americans: How Much, and Who Pays?" In *Hidden Costs, Values Lost: Uninsurance in America,* reviewed by Hugh H. Tilson and Joseph P. Newhouse, 38-61. Washington, DC: National Academies Press, 2003. https://www.ncbi.nlm.nih.gov/books/NBK221653/.

McWhinney, James. "Medicare vs. Medicaid: What's the Difference?" *Investopedia.* Last modified April 15, 2020. https://www.investopedia.com/articles/personal-finance/081114/medicaid-vs-medicare.asp.

Price, Sterling. "Average Cost of Health Insurance (2020)." Value-Penguin. Last modified October 12, 2020. https://www.value-penguin.com/average-cost-of-health-insurance.

Sherry Glied. Interview by KQED. *Healthcare Crisis: Who's at Risk?* PBS, (2000). https://www.pbs.org/healthcarecrisis/Exprts_intrvw/s_glied.htm.

Tappe, Anneken. "Nearly 43 Million Americans Have Filed for Unemployment Benefits during the Pandemic." CNN. Cable News Network. Last modified June 4, 2020. https://www.cnn.com/2020/06/04/economy/unemployment-benefits-corona-virus/index.html.

Tolbert, Jennifer, Kendal Orger, Natalie Singer, and Anthony Damico. *Key Facts About the Uninsured Population.* Issue Brief. Henry J. Kaiser Family Foundation, 2019. Accessed October 21, 2020. https://www.kff.org/uninsured/issue-brief/key-facts-about-the-uninsured-population/.

U.S. Centers for Medicare & Medicaid Services. "History." CMS. Accessed October 21, 2020. https://www.cms.gov/About-CMS/Agency-Information/History.

U.S. Centers for Medicare & Medicaid Services. "What's Medicare?" Medicare. Accessed October 21, 2020. https://www.medicare.gov/what-medicare-covers/your-medicare-coverage-choices/whats-medicare.

Uwe E. Reinhardt. Interview by KQED. *Healthcare Crisis: Who's at Risk?* PBS, (2000). https://www.pbs.org/healthcarecrisis/Exprts_intrvw/u_reinhardt.htm.

CHAPTER 7

"Eighth Broadband Progress Report." Federal Communications Commission. Federal Communications Commission. Last modified August 23, 2012. https://www.fcc.gov/reports-research/reports/broadband-progress-reports/eighth-broadband-progress-report.

Lacktman, Nathaniel M. "New Massachusetts Bills Propose Telehealth Insurance Coverage, Practice Standards." *Health Care Law Today (blog), Foley & Lardner LLP*, March 20, 2019. https://www.foley.com/en/insights/publications/2019/03/new-massachusetts-bills-propose-telehealth-insuran.

"My Record." Will Haskell 2020. Will Haskell for CT, 2020. https://www.willhaskell.com/my-record.

Nesbitt, Thomas S. "The Evolution of Telehealth: Where Have We Been and Where Are We Going?" In *The Role of Telehealth in an Evolving Health Care Environment: Workshop Summary*, edited by Tracy A. Lustig, 11–16. Washington, DC: National Academies Press, 2012. https://www.ncbi.nlm.nih.gov/books/NBK207141/.

Patel, Nilay and Makena Kelly. "Sen. Ed Markey on the Politics of Technology." June 16, 2020. In *The Vergecast*. Podcast, MP3 audio, 57:08. https://www.theverge.com/2020/6/16/21291652/senator-ed-markey-interview-broadband-access-net-neutrality-contract-tracing-vergecast.

Roth, Mandy. "New Telehealth Legislation Seeks to Expand Medicare Coverage." *HealthLeaders*, October 31, 2019. https://www.

healthleadersmedia.com/innovation/new-telehealth-legisla-tion-seeks-expand-medicare-coverage.

"Telehealth Services." U.S. Senator Brian Schatz of Hawaii. Last modified April 29, 2020. https://www.schatz.senate.gov/coro-navirus/health/telehealth.

V.A. General Assembly. Senate. *Telemedicine Services; originating site.* SB5087. 2020 Special Session 1. https://www.richmondsun-light.com/bill/2020/sb5087/fulltext/.

Wicklund, Eric. "Congressional Support Builds for Broadband Funding to Aid Telehealth." *mHealth Intelligence.* Last mod-ified May 22, 2020. https://mhealthintelligence.com/news/congressional-support-builds-for-broadband-funding-to-aid-telehealth.

CHAPTER 8

"Avera ECARE Telemedicine." Avera eCARE Telemedicine Experts. Avera Health. Accessed October 21, 2020. https://www.averae-care.org/ecare/.

"Fera's Story: Avera ECARE Provides Immediate Intervention after ATV Turnover." Avera Health. Last modified August 31, 2016. https://www.avera.org/balance/telemedicine/feras-story-ave-ra-ecare-provides-immediate-intervention-after-at/.

"History." A Brief History of Telehealth at MUSC. Medical Uni-versity of South Carolina. Accessed October 21, 2020. https://muschealth.org/medical-services/telehealth/about/history.

Meyers, Linsey. "Telemedicine—The Answer to Rural Medicine Challenges | Linsey Meyers | TEDxUSD." TEDx Talks. Uploaded March 29, 2017. YouTube video, 14:23. https://www.youtube.com/watch?v=7O2tQTRjzJo.

The U.S. Census Bureau. "City and Town Population Totals: 2010-2019." United States Department of Commerce. Last modified March 24, 2020, https://www.census.gov/data/tables/time-series/demo/popest/2010s-total-cities-and-towns.html.

"Westby, Montana." Westby, Montana (MT 59275) profile: population, maps, real estate, averages, homes, statistics, relocation, travel, jobs, hospitals, schools, crime, moving, houses, news, sex offenders. Accessed October 21, 2020. http://www.city-data.com/city/Westby-Montana.html.

CHAPTER 9

"About Amwell." Amwell. American Well. Accessed October 21, 2020. https://business.amwell.com/about-us.

"AI-Enabled Mental Health Treatment Platform Goes Live: Ieso Digital Health." Ieso. Ieso Digital Health. Accessed October 21, 2020. https://www.iesohealth.com/en-gb/news/world-s-first-ai-enabled-mental-health-treatment-platform-goes-live.

Alltucker, Kenneth. "USA Today: 'Really Astonishing': Average Cost of Hospital ER Visit Surges 176% in a Decade, Report Says." HCCI. Health Care Cost Institute. Last modified June 4, 2019. https://healthcostinstitute.org/in-the-news/usa-today.

Curry, Kerry. "The Doctor Will Text You Now." *D CEO*, March, 2018. https://www.dmagazine.com/publications/d-ceo/2018/march/ieso-digital-health-dan-clark/.

"How Much Does an Online Doctor Visit on Amwell Cost?" Amwell. American Well. Accessed October 21, 2020. https://amwell.com/cm/faq/how-much-does-an-online-doctor-visit-on-amwell-cost/.

"Is My Online Doctor Visit Private and Secure?" Amwell. American Well. Accessed October 21, 2020. https://amwell.com/cm/faq/is-my-online-doctor-visit-private-and-secure/.

Salleh, Fariza. "Singapore Telemedicine Startup Doctor Anywhere Thrives as Virtual Healthcare Becomes the New Normal." *Business Insider*. Insider Inc. Last modified September 30, 2020. https://www.businessinsider.com/singapore-telemedicine-startup-doctor-anywhere-thrives-in-new-normal-2020-9.

"Types of Mental Health Problems We Treat: Ieso Digital Health." Ieso Digital Health. Accessed October 21, 2020. https://www.iesohealth.com/en-gb/what-we-treat.